Evidence-based Practice for Occupational Therapists

Evidence-based Practice for Occupational Therapists

M. Clare Taylor

Blackwell
Science

Editorial Offices:
Blackwell Science Ltd, 9600 Garsington Road, Oxford OX4 2DQ, UK
Tel: +44 (0)1865 776868
Blackwell Publishing Inc., 350 Main Street, Malden, MA 02148-5020, USA
Tel: +1 781 388 8250
Blackwell Science Asia Pty, 550 Swanston Street, Carlton, Victoria 3053, Australia
Tel: +61 (0)3 8359 1011

First published 2000
Reprinted 2001, 2002, 2004

Library of Congress Cataloging-in-Publication Data
Taylor, M. Clare.
Evidence-based practice for occupational therapists/M. Clare Taylor.
p. ; cm.
Includes bibliographical references and index.
ISBN 0-632-05177-9 (pb)
1. Occupational therapy. 2. Evidence- based medicine. I. Title.
[DNLM: 1. Occupational Therapy—organization & administration.
2. Evidence-Based Medicine.
WB 555 T244 2000]
RM735.6 .T39 2000
615.8′2—dc21

99-088122

ISBN 0-632-05177-9

A catalogue record for this title is available from the British Library

Set in 11/15pt Souvenir Light
by DP Photosetting, Aylesbury, Bucks
Printed and bound in Great Britain
by The Alden Press, Oxford

The publisher's policy is to use permanent paper from mills that operate a sustainable forestry policy, and which has been manufactured from pulp processed using acid-free and elementary chlorine-free practices. Furthermore, the publisher ensures that the text paper and cover board used have met acceptable environmental accreditation standards.

For further information on Blackwell Publishing, visit our website:
www.blackwellpublishing.com

To the memory of my parents,
Charles and Audrey Taylor

CONTENTS

ACKNOWLEDGEMENTS

A number of people have helped with the evolution and writing of this book. Particular recognition and thanks are due to: Sally Croft, Librarian, Dorset House, Oxford Brookes University for her skills and knowledge of resources and literature available to OTs; and to my colleagues and friends within the School of Health Care, Oxford Brookes University for their critical comments and proof-reading of the manuscript, and for providing the ideas for some of the scenarios used in the book.

Chapter 1
INTRODUCTION

Evidence-based practice appears to be one of the buzzwords (or buzz terms) of current health and social care practice. But what *is* evidence-based practice, where did the term come from and how can it help overworked occupational therapists (OT – OT is an abbreviation that can be used to mean both occupational therapist, as here, or occupational therapy. Both meanings are used in this book but spelt out in full should there be potential for confusion) to make decisions about the effectiveness of their practice? This chapter will attempt to answer these questions.

The chapter begins by defining the term 'evidence-based practice' and then outlining the background to, and the necessity for, an evidence-based approach to occupational therapy (OT) practice. There is often confusion over what is 'research', what is 'audit' and what is 'evidence-based practice.' This chapter will attempt to clarify the differences between these three approaches to finding and using information to improve practice. Having established what evidence-based practice is, and what it is not, the chapter will then outline the process; in other words, how to implement evidence-based practice. The nature of evidence will be discussed and the chapter will conclude with an overview of how to use this book as a practical guide to evidence-based practice.

What is evidence-based practice?

The term 'evidence-based *medicine*' was coined at McMaster University medical school in the 1980s as a way of describing a process of problem-based clinical teaching and learning that involved students and clinicians in searching for, and evaluating, the evidence for clinical practice (Bennett *et al.*, 1987; Shin *et al.*, 1993). Its philosophical origins, however, can be found in mid-19th century Paris (Sackett *et al.*, 1996; Rangachari, 1997) where Pierre Charles Alexandre Louis used statistical analysis to demonstrate that blood letting had no value as a clinical intervention.

Sackett *et al.* (1996: 71) have defined evidence-based medicine as:

> 'the conscientious, explicit and judicious use of current best evidence in making decisions about the care of individual patients.'

Although evidence-based *medicine* is still a commonly used term, the evidence-based process has broadened and evolved and now evidence-based *practice* is seen as a more appropriate term.

The concern most frequently expressed about evidence-based practice is that it will become prescriptive and will lead to cost cutting and 'cook-book' practice (Sackett *et al.*, 1996) where there is one recognised, cheap, intervention for a specific problem. In OT this would mean a return to the days of *Refer to Occupational Therapy* (Shopland *et al.*, 1975), that neat, pocket-sized book which listed all the things the basic grade OT needed to know in order to be able to treat any stroke, head injury or total hip, etc. Sackett *et al.* (1996) argued strongly that evidence-based practice is only a part of the clinical decision-making process and that any judgements and clinical decisions are based on a mix of clinical expertise and the best evidence. The aim is to ensure that the interventions used are the most effective and the safest options. External evidence is just one strand of the process and must be blended with clinical judgement and patient preference.

The essence of evidence-based practice is that the decision process is explicit and therefore clearly articulated so that decisions can be explained to the patient/client and justified to colleagues and managers. Evidence is gathered conscientiously but it is used judiciously so that the experience of the OT, the needs of the patient/client, the demands of the system and the up-to-date best evidence are weighed together in order that the best care is given. Evidence-based practice is just one of the tools of clinical reasoning and reflective practice. However, because of the use of up-to-date best evidence, evidence-based practice is a powerful tool.

The background to evidence-based practice

Gray (1997) proposed that the management of health care, over the last three decades, had developed from the principles of efficiency and quality. Efficiency can be translated into 'doing things cheaply', whilst quality can be translated as 'doing things better'. This has led to a management philosophy of 'doing things right'. This, however, has not always meant using the 'right' or the 'best' intervention. This may sometimes be in conflict with the health and social care practitioner's philosophy of doing the right thing, in other words doing 'good' instead of 'harm'. Whilst health and social care practice has attempted to do 'good' and the 'right' thing, it has not always been possible to argue that the 'right' intervention is based on anything other than common sense. Cochrane (1972) highlighted medicine's collective ignorance of the effects and effectiveness of health care. He proposed that less than 15% of all medical interventions were based on clear clinical trials of effectiveness.

Gray (1997) argued that the philosophy of health care management for the 21st century will be 'doing the right things right' and that this will mean making decisions about interventions which are based on good evidence and which may have a profound effect on the nature of clinical practice. Research and practice need to be drawn together so that practice is underpinned by sound evidence, and so that clinicians can demonstrate to service managers that they are 'doing the right things right' (Gray, 1997: 20). The problem for OTs, very often, is defining and measuring what 'good' and 'sound' evidence actually means.

Comparison of research, audit and evidence-based practice

The terms 'research', 'audit' and 'evidence-based practice' are liberally used within the health care literature, but how well do practitioners understand exactly what the different terms mean. This section will attempt to tease out the differences and similarities between research, audit and evidence-based practice.

Defining the terms

'Research' has been defined as:

> 'a systematic process of gathering and synthesising empirical data so as to generate knowledge about a given population for a selected topic' (Bailey, 1991: 1).

Whilst 'audit' has been defined as:

> 'the systematic critical analysis of the quality of medical care, including the procedures used in diagnosis and treatment, the use of resources and the resulting outcome and quality of life for the patient' (Sale, 1996: 71).

Finally, as stated earlier, 'evidence-based practice' has been defined as:

> 'the conscientious, explicit and judicious use of current best evidence in making decisions about the care of individuals' (Sackett *et al*., 1996: 71).

Similarities and differences

There are many similarities between research, audit and evidence-based practice. There are also some crucial differences. These are summarised in Table 1.1.

Research, audit and evidence-based practice are all *systematic* processes for finding information to improve and refine interventions and practice. But, whilst research aims to generate new knowledge, both audit and evidence-based practice use existing practice and existing knowledge to review and improve interventions. Audit uses existing practice and evidence-based practice uses existing knowledge as the focus of the review process.

Table 1.1 Similarities and differences of research, audit and evidence-based practice.

Research	Audit	Evidence-based practice
Systematic investigation to increase the sum of knowledge	Systematic approach to identify possible improvements and mechanisms to bring them about	Systematic review of evidence to guide clinical interventions
Aims to identify the most effective form of treatment	Aims to compare actual performance against agreed standards of practice	Aims to use evidence to underpin clinical decision making
Results extend to the general population	Results apply only to the population examined	Results apply to a particular problem, intervention and outcome
May be a one-off study	The process is ongoing and continuous	Philosophy for decision making
Data collection is complex, new data being collected	Data collection is via records and follow-up of patients	Data is drawn from existing research

The outcomes of research may change practice throughout the world whilst the outcomes of audit may change practice within one particular setting. The outcomes of evidence-based practice, however, may influence the interventions used with one person, within one department, or at a regional or national level if clinical guidelines are developed.

Research is about generating evidence, audit is about assessing practice, and evidence-based practice is about putting evidence into current practice. As already mentioned, Gray (1997: 20) talks about evidence-based practice as 'doing the right things right'. Research is used to tell us what the right things are, audit tells us if we are doing the things that we are doing right, and evidence-based practice draws these two strands together to help the clinician to use the right intervention properly.

The OT process is essentially the same as the processes of

research, audit and evidence-based practice in that a problem needs to be identified, an intervention must be planned and carried out, and the outcome must be assessed and evaluated.

The need for an evidence-based approach to practice

As OTs, in order to survive in the current health and social care climate, we need to demonstrate that our interventions are both clinically and cost effective. But where do we find the evidence to support our claims to clinical and cost effectiveness? As Table 1.2 illustrates, the range of published literature available which *might* contain the evidence for practice is vast and ever growing.

This list is by no means exhaustive. Nor does it include what is known as 'grey' literature. This is literature that has been published or is in the public domain but does not have an International Standard Book Number (ISBN) in the case of a book or an International Standard Serial Number (ISSN) in the case of a serial publication such as a journal and is, therefore, not easily accessed from databases. Grey literature includes: theses and dissertations, which are held in university and departmental libraries; conference presentations and proceedings, which may not be fully reported or published; and all manner of other material on research and projects which has been written up but goes no further than a library shelf. Occupational therapists in the UK are now being educated at degree level. They are all spending long hours researching and writing dissertations and yet few of these will be published or become available to a wider audience. Whilst many of these, on well-worn topics such as:

- How nurses/doctors/GPs/the Multi-disciplinary team (MDT) view the role of OT
- The role of OT within mental health

may not be of great value to a wider audience. Some, for example:

- *Homophobia amongst OT students: Issues, Incidence and Implications* (Haddon-Silver, 1993)

Table 1.2 Journals with the potential for providing the evidence base for OT interventions.

Access by Design
American Journal of Occupational Therapy
American Journal of Physical Medicine and Rehabilitation
Archives of Physical Medicine and Rehabilitation
Australian Occupational Therapy Journal
British Journal of Learning Disabilities
British Journal of Occupational Therapy
British Journal of Therapy and Rehabilitation
Canadian Journal of Occupational Therapy
Clinical Rehabilitation
Disability and Rehabilitation
Disability and Society
Evidence-based Mental Health
Health Service Journal
International Journal of Rehabilitation Research
Irish Occupational Therapy Journal
Israeli Journal of Occupational Therapy
Journal of Allied Health
Journal of Applied Research in Intellectual Abilities
Journal of Evaluation in Clinical Practice
Journal of Hand Therapy
Journal of Interprofessional Care
Journal of Occupational Science – Australia
Journal of Rehabilitation Research and Development
Neuropsychology Rehabilitation
New Zealand Journal of Occupational Therapy
Occupational Therapy in Health Care
Occupational Therapy in Mental Health
Occupational Therapy International
Occupational Therapy Journal of Research
OT Practice
Physical and Occupational Therapy in Geriatrics
Physical and Occupational Therapy in Pediatrics
Scandinavian Journal of Rehabilitation Medicine
Social Science and Medicine
South African Journal of Occupational Therapy

- *Does the Rivermead Extended ADL Score Indicate a Patient's Level of Independence after Discharge?* (Cooper, 1995)
- *Do OT Students Consider Sexual Orientation When Implementing Treatment?* (Littlewood, 1997)
- *An Audit of the Reliability of the Frenchay Activities Index* (Piercy, 1998)

provide useful evidence and deserve to be available. The College of Occupational Therapists' (COT) Library does hold copies of many Masters and Doctoral theses produced by OTs. However, too much valuable OT evidence remains as grey literature.

How can the busy OT hope to keep up to date with all the possible sources of evidence? This is why an evidence-based approach to practice is needed. Evidence-based practice provides OTs with a systematic framework for reviewing the evidence to underpin their practice. Sackett (1997) has shown that, in the majority of cases, an evidence-based approach does not, in fact, change the intervention decision. What evidence-based practice does, however, is give OTs the tools and the evidence to justify that intervention to themselves, the patient/client and the management.

The process of evidence-based practice

Evidence-based practice is a process which is essentially the same as both the research process and the OT process. All of these processes are based on a number of stages, which include:

- Identify a problem
- Plan/design an intervention/action
- Carry out the intervention/action
- Evaluate the process and the outcome

Rosenberg and Donald (1995) have identified four stages to the evidence-based practice process. These four stages are:

- Formulate a clear clinical question from the patient's problem
- Search the literature for relevant clinical articles/evidence
- Evaluate (critically appraise) this evidence for its validity and usefulness
- Implement useful findings in clinical practice

Having established what the patient's/client's problems are, evidence-based practice can be initiated by asking 'clinical' questions related to diagnosis, prognosis, treatment, iatrogenic harm, quality of care and health economics (Rosenberg & Donald, 1995). The questions should focus on the problem, the intervention and the outcome. Evidence-based questions are usually articulated in terms of:

> *What is the evidence for the effectiveness of* **x** *(the intervention) for* **y** *(the outcome in a patient with* **z** *(the problem or diagnosis)?*

This might fit very nicely into medical practice when thinking about whether treatment with aspirin and warfarin will reduce the risk of stroke in an elderly lady with hypertension, but how can it relate to the complexities of OT practice? However, with the basic OT skill of creative thinking, it is perfectly possible to focus on a problem, an intervention and an outcome and, thus, initiate evidence-based practice.

Each stage of the process will be explored in this book. Asking and formulating a 'clear clinical question from the patient's problem' will be discussed below. The three remaining stages of finding, appraising and using evidence will form the basis of the remaining chapters.

Asking useful questions

The first stage in the search for evidence to underpin practice is to ask a clear question. This question will be used to guide the search for evidence and so must be clear and specific, otherwise a vast amount of evidence may be found that has little, if any, relevance to the initial question. A great deal of time can be wasted down the interesting side-tracks this may produce. However, getting side-tracked will not answer the original question and may reinforce negative assumptions about the value, or lack of value, of an evidence-based approach to practice.

As outlined above, a useful question consists of:

- A problem
- An intervention
- An outcome

In other words, you must identify: 'who', i.e. a patient or client group; a particular occupational or clinical problem; 'what', i.e. the intervention you think might be of value for this problem; and, finally, 'why', i.e. the outcome or reason for using the intervention. Without the outcome the question can become vague and woolly and any evidence found will have limited value in answering the question. The more time you spend formulating your question the easier the task of finding the right evidence specific to your needs will be.

Some authors (Richardson *et al.*, 1995) have argued that a 'well-built' question should include not just an intervention but also a comparative intervention. This is common practice when looking at treatment interventions within a medical context. This comparative approach may have relevance to some OT evidence-based practitioners, however for many OT problems comparison of interventions may not be appropriate or useful.

Richardson *et al.* (1995) referred to the elements of the question

Table 1.3 Elements of a well-built evidence-based question.

Problem	Intervention	Comparative intervention	Outcome
Describe your patient/client and her/his problem. This may be a diagnosis or a functional or occupational performance problem. The description should also include all key information e.g. age, sex, occupational status	Describe the main intervention	*if applicable* Describe the comparative or alternative intervention. This may also take the form of alternative approaches to the intervention e.g. group or individual sessions; different frequency of intervention	Describe what you hope to achieve or what effect the intervention may have on your patient/client

(the problem, the outcome, the intervention/comparison) as the 'anatomy' of an evidence-based question. As we will see in Chapter 2 on finding the evidence, the clearer you are about each element of the question and the components of each element, the more successful you will be in finding evidence and answering your question. Table 1.3 outlines the four elements of an evidence-based question.

Practical applications of this process will now be discussed. Client scenarios will be used to create evidence-based questions. These scenarios and questions will be used in later chapters to illustrate the application of evidence-based practice for OT.

After the scenario is described, the problem, intervention and outcome will be highlighted and an evidence-based question will be developed.

Client scenario 1

You are the OT manager for a mental health Trust. You are beginning to explore evidence-based practice and are wondering how an evidence-based approach might be applied to your service. Because of economic and service constraints you are reviewing the value and effectiveness of a number of OT interventions and areas of practice. You are particularly concerned about the value of some of the activity groups within the main OT department. Rather than focusing on one particular activity you decide to adopt a broad evidence-based approach. You decide to explore the concept of 'activity' within a specific diagnostic and symptom context. The majority of clients who attend the various activity groups have some level of depression.

Problem	*Intervention*	*Outcome*
Depression	Activity	Improved mood

What is the evidence for the value of activity as a means of improving mood in clients with depression?

Client scenario 2

Recently you have been running a horticulture group as part of the activity programme for the eating disorders unit you work on.

The group has proved to be remarkably successful. You are keen to carry out some research into the value of horticulture as a purposeful activity, but are unsure about how to start this research. You decide to carry out an evidence-based review of the value of horticulture as a purposeful activity as a way of helping to develop your research ideas.

Problem	*Intervention*	*Outcome*
Eating disorders: • anorexia • bulimia	Horticulture	Improve self-esteem: • increase confidence in self • increase confidence in abilities

What is the evidence for the value of horticulture as a purposeful activity and means of improving self-esteem and confidence in clients with eating disorders?

Client scenario 3

You have recently been appointed to a post which includes a unit specialising in the care of people who are human immuno-deficiency virus (HIV) positive or who have acquired immuno-deficiency syndrome (AIDS). You are exploring potential areas of OT intervention. You notice that many of the clients appear to be experiencing high levels of anxiety which limits their occupational performance. You have also read that levels of anxiety may affect the body's immune responses. You feel that an area of OT intervention might be in anxiety management. However, before embarking on designing an anxiety management programme you decide to explore whether this is an effective intervention and what evidence exists to support your proposal for establishing anxiety management as part of the OT intervention on the unit.

Problem	*Intervention*	*Outcome*
Anxiety in clients with HIV/AIDS	Anxiety management	Improved function and occupational performance; improved immunity; improved quality of life

What is the evidence for the value of anxiety management as a means of improving function/occupational performance/ immunity/quality of life in clients who are HIV positive or who have AIDS?

Client scenario 4

You have been running an out-patient group and course on joint protection and energy conservation for clients with rheumatoid arthritis (RA). The energy conservation aspect of the groups seems to be particularly successful. You are preparing a proposal to extend the energy conservation group to include other clients who experience periods of fatigue, such as people with multiple sclerosis (MS) or AIDS. You decide to explore the evidence base for using energy conservation education as a way of decreasing fatigue within these client groups. You are also interested to explore whether group or individual sessions are more effective or whether sessions should focus solely on information or should include discussion and a self-help focus.

Problem	*Intervention*	*Alternative interventions*	*Outcome*
Fatigue associated with: • MS • HIV/AIDS • RA	Energy conservation	Individual or group session; length of course; handouts and/ or discussion; self-help	Improved quality of life; increased occupational performance; decreased fatigue

What is the evidence for the value of energy conservation as a means of improving quality of life/occupational performance and decreasing levels of fatigue in clients who experience high levels of fatigue associated with chronic illnesses such as MS, AIDS, RA?

Client scenario 5

As a final year OT student you are expected to carry out either a piece of empirical research or a systematic review of the literature pertinent to an area of OT practice. One of your fieldwork placements was spent at a specialist rehabilitation unit for people following brain injury. Whilst you were at the unit you noticed that many of the clients had memory impairments. The approach used with these clients was to give each client a variety of memory aids. Working with a number of clients, you had begun to explore alternative approaches such as using activities and groups as well as aids and education to improve memory function. You decide, for your final year project, to carry out a systematic review of the evidence into the effectiveness of a number of approaches to improving memory function.

Problem	*Intervention*	*Alternative interventions*	*Outcome*
Memory impairment following brain injury	Memory aids	Group or individual sessions; education or activity	Decrease in confusion; increase in memory function; increase in occupational performance

What is the evidence for the value of memory aids as a means of decreasing confusion and improving memory function and occupational performance in clients with memory impairment as a result of brain injury?

Whilst some of these questions may appear vague, the aim for all of these questions and scenarios is to use them as tools to illustrate the practical application of evidence-based practice for OTs. The scenarios and questions aim to cover a broad spectrum of OT practice. However, the author acknowledges that it is not practical to explore the totality of OT interventions within one small text.

Levels of evidence

Whilst all research can provide evidence upon which to judge the usefulness of an intervention, some evidence is seen as stronger, more rigorous or more valid than others. When looking for the 'best' evidence, some evidence is seen as better than others. Within evidence-based practice there is a hierarchy, or levels, of 'best' evidence. Table 1.4 outlines the hierarchy of evidence. The origin of this hierarchy is in the work of Fletcher and Sackett (Canadian Task Force on the Periodic Health Examination, 1979) whilst current discussion of levels of evidence can be found on http://www.cebm.jr2.ox.ac.uk/docs/levels.html

It is important to remember that these levels of evidence have been developed within a medical context which makes limited acknowledgement of the value of qualitative research.

Table 1.4 Levels of evidence

- Systematic reviews and meta-analyses of randomised controlled trials
- Randomised controlled trials
- Non-randomised experimental studies
- Non-experimental studies
- Respected opinion, expert discussion

The most powerful and the most rigorous evidence can be found in systematic reviews and meta-analyses. This is where all the available published and unpublished evidence has been reviewed and synthesised and the findings of this re-analysis are presented. The strength of systematic review lies in the vast numbers of subjects and, therefore, the range of data, which have been drawn together.

This frequently results in findings which become highly significant findings or can result in statistically significant findings, where previously the research had shown results that were not, in themselves, statistically significant, or where the level of significance of individual trials is small.

The evidence which is drawn together in a systematic review tends to come from randomised controlled trials (RCTs). Randomised controlled trials are often seen as the 'gold standard' in terms of rigorous evidence. For some, RCT evidence is the only evidence worth considering when reviewing the effectiveness of an intervention. Non-randomised experimental studies include controlled clinical trials (CCTs). These are also seen as valuable sources of evidence and are included in the Cochrane Trials Register. Controlled clinical trials are where two groups are compared but allocation to the treatment or the non-treatment group is not randomly carried out.

Non-experimental studies and descriptive studies are seen as providing weak evidence, which has limited validity. Non-experimental studies include single-subject design research and studies using pre-test/post-test designs or where one cohort of clients is assessed both prior to intervention and after intervention. Descriptive studies include surveys and qualitative research. The lowest level of evidence is expert opinion and discussion.

The limited value and credibility given to non-experimental and descriptive evidence presents us, as OTs, with a problem. The focus of much of the research within OT has tended to be descriptive and qualitative. However, the value of rigorous qualitative research is being acknowledged, with evidence-based gurus such as David Sackett (1997) accepting that the nature of 'best' evidence may depend upon the question that has been asked and that for some investigations good qualitative research may, indeed, provide the best available evidence. The goal of any evidence-based practitioner should be to find evidence at the highest level first and then to explore evidence lower down the hierarchy. The strength and validity of any evidence should always be clearly stated when using evidence to underpin the effectiveness of any intervention.

How to use this book

The main aim of this book is to make evidence-based practice accessible to OTs. The scenarios and questions outlined in this chapter will be used later in the book as practical illustrations of finding, appraising and using evidence to review the effectiveness of OT interventions and practice. Each chapter will also include activities to help you to consolidate your evidence-based practice skills.

The rest of the book will explore each stage of the evidence-based practice process in turn; beginning with finding the evidence, then looking at appraising various types of research evidence (RCTs, systematic reviews and qualitative research) before considering how evidence-based practice might work in OT practice settings. The book concludes by giving an annotated listing of a variety of resources that might be helpful to the evidence-based practitioner. Whilst the flow of the book follows the stages of the evidence-based practice process, it is the author's intention that each chapter can stand alone and can be read separately, and that when you have finished working through this book you should have a clear and practical grasp of how an evidence-based approach can help OTs to explore and evaluate the effectiveness of their practice.

Activity

- Take a client/patient or scenario from your practice
- Look at the client/scenario in terms of the elements of evidence-based practice, namely
  - ☐ Problem
  - ☐ Intervention
  - ☐ Outcome
- Outline the components of each of these elements for your client/scenario
- Write an evidence-based question, using the elements you have identified

Further reading

The following references will be useful for the reader who wishes to explore the background to evidence-based practice further, or who wishes to explore wider issues within the remit of evidence-based practice.

British Journal of Therapy and Rehabilitation (1996) Supplement on evidence-based practice and mental health. *British Journal of Therapy and Rehabilitation*, **3**(12), 659–70.

Canadian Association of Occupational Therapists (1998) Special edition on evidence-based practice. *Canadian Journal of Occupational Therapy*, **65**(3).

College of Occupational Therapists (1997). Special edition on evidence-based practice. *British Journal of Occupational Therapy*, **60**(11).

Gray, J.A.M. (1997) *Evidence-based Healthcare*. Edinburgh: Churchill Livingstone.

Hope, T. (1997) *Evidence-based Patient Choice*. London: King's Fund.

Lockett, T. (1997), *Evidence-based and Cost-effective Medicine for the Uninitiated*. Oxford: Radcliffe Medical Press.

Rosenberg, W. & Donald, A. (1995) Evidence based medicine: an approach to clinical problem-solving. *British Medical Journal*, **310**, 1122–6.

Sackett, D.L., Richardson, W.S., Rosenberg, W. & Hayes, R.B. (1997) *Evidence-based Medicine: How to Practice and Teach EBM*. New York: Churchill Livingstone.

Sackett, D.L., Rosenberg, W.M.C., Gray, J.A.M., Haynes, R.B. & Richardson, W.S. (1996) Evidence-based medicine: what it is and what it isn't. *British Medical Journal*, **312**, 71–2.

Chapter 2
FINDING THE EVIDENCE

Having decided to adopt an evidence-based approach to practice and having developed an evidence-based question, the next stage in the process is to attempt to find the evidence. Having found the evidence you will need to appraise it. This will be considered in Chapters 3–5. This chapter will concentrate on the process of searching for and finding the evidence. The chapter will begin by reviewing the potential sources of evidence that are available to the evidence-based practitioner. The process of searching will then be outlined and the scenarios and problems outlined in Chapter 1 will be developed and used to illustrate the successes and pitfalls of searching. The various searches will also use a variety of databases and sources of material to allow the reader to compare the potential usefulness of a range of resources. Having found the references and citations of evidence it is important to be able to access and get hold of the material. The chapter will conclude by discussing ways of accessing and then storing evidence. The chapter will also include a number of activities for readers to consolidate their evidence-based skills.

Sources of evidence

We noted in Chapter 1 that there was a hierarchy of evidence:

- Systematic reviews and meta-analyses of randomised controlled trials (RCTs)
- Randomised controlled trials

- Non-randomised experimental studies
- Non-experimental studies
- Descriptive studies
- Respected opinion, expert discussion

The next question to ask is where can the evidence-based OT find any of this evidence? Evidence can be gathered from a range of sources, including:

- Observations
- Discussion with colleagues
- Clients
- Conferences
- Books
- Journal articles

But which of these are sources of the 'best' evidence?

The hierarchy of evidence begins to help identify the sources to tap first and indicates that the best evidence will be found in the results of RCTs and systematic reviews of RCTs. The next question is where best to access good quality RCT-based information. Research information can be found in conference proceedings, books and journals. But which of these will provide the 'best' and most up-to-date information?

Conferences, books or journals?

Common sense might lead us to think that conferences would be the best sources of good quality, up-to-date research evidence. However, this is not necessarily the case. Conferences are certainly sources of up-to-date and current evidence. Presenters will often be talking about work still in progress or recently completed. However, a conference will not always be the source of the best quality information. Conference presentations are usually subjected to relatively low-level quality filters. The conference committee will review and choose papers for presentation based on a number of criteria. One of these criteria may be the rigour of the research, but other factors will also influence decisions about inclusion of papers. Conferences and conference proceedings should be viewed as useful sources of contact with experts and ideas about current developments in the field but should not be seen as sources of high-quality evidence.

Books should also be viewed with caution. The major problem with books is that they are dated almost as soon as they are published. The process of getting a book from idea to print can take, in the worst of cases, several years by which time knowledge may have moved on. A frequently cited example from the world of evidence-based *medicine* is the evidence for the use of thrombolytic therapy with patients who have had heart attacks. The RCT evidence was available in 1970 and yet it was not until the late 1980s, some 15 to 17 years later, that the medical textbooks routinely recommended the use of thrombolytic therapy for patients who had experienced heart attacks (Gray, 1997). The evidence might be available, but books may not be the best place to begin a search for *current* best evidence.

The 'best' and most current evidence will be found in journals. However, some journals are 'better' than others. Some journals contain articles that have been rigorously peer reviewed, whilst other journals are less rigorous in their approach. The peer review process attempts to ensure that only good-quality research is published. Reviewers will comment not only on the applicability and readability of the article but also on the rigour of the research design, the robustness of the analysis and the validity of the conclusions being drawn. Journal articles will also include an overview of the methods used in the research and, thus, allow the reader to critically appraise the quality of the research and its evidence. Journals should provide the major source of good-quality evidence for the evidence-based OT.

Indexes and databases

Having identified journals as the best sources of evidence, how does the evidence-based OT find the right articles in the right journals?

The novice searcher often goes into a library, finds a likely looking journal and starts flicking through it in the hope of finding something useful. However, with some 20 OT-specific journals and over 20 000 journals published annually (Mulrow, 1994), this is not the best approach for the evidence-based OT. Searching should be systematic and focused.

Bibliographic indexes and databases have been developed to help readers and researchers locate the most suitable information for particular topics. Databases provide access to information from large numbers of journals (and books, in some cases). Subject headings are used to code and cross-reference each entry so that, by choosing key words, the evidence-based OT can search for the most relevant information for the topic or question. Databases tend to be available in both hard-copy format or on CD-ROM. Some databases are also available on-line via the Internet. Chapter 7 contains detailed information on the most appropriate databases for the evidence-based OT. These databases are:

General databases

- AMED
- ASSIA
- BIDS
- CINAHL
- EMBASE
- ERIC
- MEDLINE
- PsychLit
- PubMed
- Sociological Abstracts

OT databases

- OTBibSys
- OTDBASE

Specialist evidence-based databases (These databases, unlike general databases, employ quality checks, and so will only include citations for work which meets their standards for good evidence.

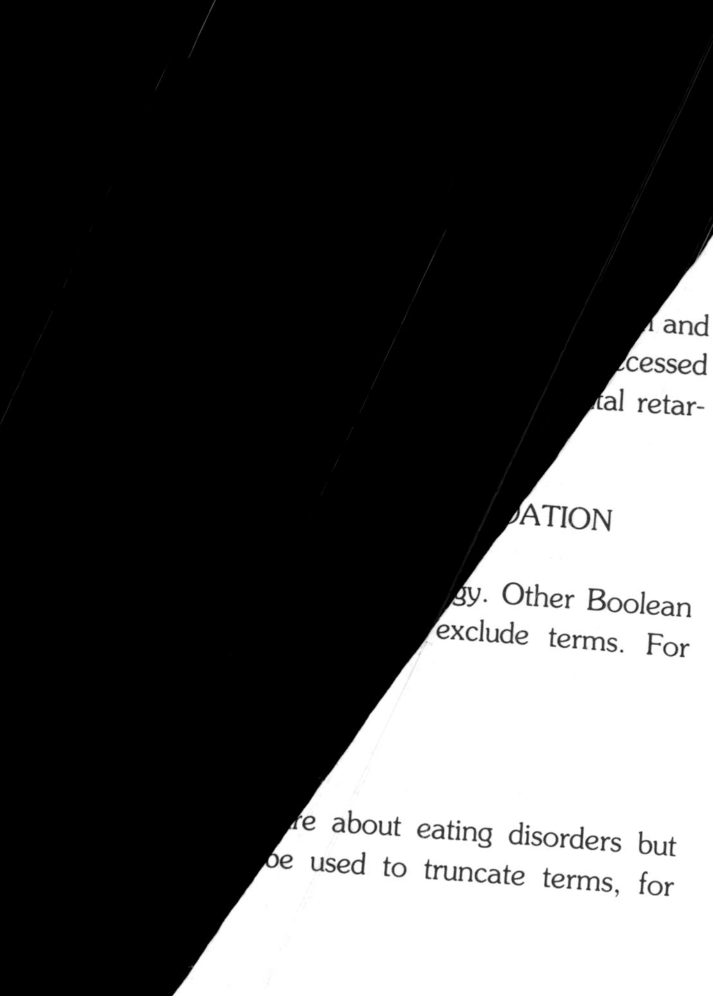

- Best Evidence
- Cochrane Library
- DARE

Databases have different areas of focus, for example EMBASE, MEDLINE, and PubMed have a very medical focus, whilst AMED and CINAHL focus more on allied health. ASSIA, PsychLit and Sociological Abstracts draw heavily on social science literature and ERIC has an educational focus. Thus, some databases will be more suitable for some questions than for others. However, the evidence-based OT must also be pragmatic. The search for evidence may also be restricted by the local availability of search resources.

Activity

- Identify what databases are available locally, in:
  - public libraries
  - hospital and health authority libraries
  - university libraries
- Identify where you might be able to access and use the Internet

Searching for evidence

The most important attributes for a successful search are to be organised, systematic and focused. Without these the search will become easily side-tracked into looking at interesting but peripheral (at best) or irrelevant (at worst) areas, or will produce vast amounts of material most of which has limited value in providing an evidence-based answer to the question.

The process of successful searching consists of four stages:

- Asking a clear question, identifying the problem, intervention, alternate intervention and outcome
- Identifying the most appropriate library, collection or information source for the question
- Selecting the database most relevant to the question

- Developing a clear search strategy with key words and s
  terms.

The development of a clear question has been already
in Chapter 1.

To identify the library or collection which will pro
information for your question, you need to consider

- Whether the search will be done by you or by so
  librarian)
- How much time, money and effort you ha
  prepared to spend
- Whether you want immediate access to th
  pared to use Inter-Library Loan to acces
- Where the focus of the question lies, is
  - intervention focused
  - focused on a specific diagnosis
  - management issues
  - research focused

How you answer these will d
might be that the local Trust li
you might want to use the
Library and Information Se
versity library. Useful guide

- Guide to Libraries and Informatio
  Health care (Dale, 1997)
- ASLIB Directory of Information Sources in the U
  (Reynard & Reynard, 1996)
- Literature Searching: Where to Go and What to Look For
  (Chartered Society of Physiotherapy, 1996)

To choose the most appropriate database, you need to consider:

- Whether the focus of the question is medical or broader

Many databases use what are known as Boolean operators to help the searcher refine the search question. Thus terms can be combined to focus the search or limits can be set on the search. **AND** and **OR** are the key combining terms. Thus a searcher interested in stress management as used by OTs would search using:

STRESS MANAGEMENT **AND** OCCUPATIONAL THERAP

whilst another searcher who wanted to make sure both Britis
American literature on people with learning disabilities was a
would remember that the Americans use the term 'me
dation' and so would search with:

LEARNING DISABILITY **OR** MENTAL RETAR

to access both sets of literature and terminolo
operators include **NOT** which is used to
example:

ANOREXIA **NOT** BULIMIA

can be used to search for literatu
specific to anorexia and * can
example:

THERAP*

will access citations cont
Many of these area
takes the scenarios
and uses them as

Examples o

indexin

search will be outlined in terms of an overview of the problem, the search terms, the choice of particular databases to be searched, an overview of the searches and a review of the outcomes of the searches.

Search 1

Question and search terms

> *What is the evidence for the value of activity as a means of improving mood in clients with depression?*

Problem	*Intervention*	*Outcome*
Depression	Activity	Improved mood

Search terms:

depression	activity	mood
	purposeful activity	
	exercise	
	rehabilitation	

Choice of databases

As the focus of this question is 'purposeful activity' which is a concept specific to OT, databases which were either OT-specific or had included a wide range of OT journals were chosen. The databases used were:

OTDBASE
AMED

Search strategy: comparing OTDBASE and AMED

OTDBASE

- As the author, in common with many OTs, was not a subscriber to OTDBASE the restricted access and miniOTDBASE through http://www.mother.com/~ktherapy/ot was used.

- The OTDBASE preview category 'vocational', which is available to non-subscribers, was chosen. This category can be linked with other key words, 'leisure' was chosen.
- This search gave 31 hits (a 'hit' is any relevant reference citation identified by the search), each hit included bibliographic information and could be expanded to give the abstract.
- miniOTDBASE was then searched.
- From the table of key words 'activity' was chosen. This gave a series of five subheadings:
  - analysis
  - crafts
  - motivation
  - research
  - selection.
- For each subheading, the number of possible hits is given plus the full citations and abstracts for the three most recent articles. For example:
  - 'research' gave three potential hits
  - 'crafts' gave 11 potential hits
  - 'motivation' gave 38 potential hits
- The key word 'mental health' was also chosen. This gave 28 subheadings, of which the most relevant were searched;
  - 'activity' gave 40 hits
  - 'depression' gave 25 hits
  - 'programme cost – effectiveness' gave three hits
  - 'programme efficacy' gave 55 hits

AMED

- The key words chosen were:
  - depression
  - activity
  - rehabilitation.
- AMED's thesaurus was used to refine the search terms.
- New search terms were identified as:
  - depression
  - depressive disorder

  - human activity
  - leisure activities.
- These were combined using the Boolean operators OR and AND to give a search of:
  - depression OR depressive disorder AND human activities OR leisure activities
- This search resulted in 98 hits.
- A second search was carried out using the search terms:
  - depression OR depressive disorder AND rehabilitation, to ensure that useful articles had not been missed.
- This search resulted in 104 hits.

Outcomes of search

The OTDBASE search produced a wide variety of OT-specific references. Of the 31 hits on the 'vocational:leisure' search, three articles could have direct relevance to the question and three, one of which is in Hebrew, might have relevance to the question. From the miniOTDBASE search, of the actual citations given (21), six had direct relevance to the topic. However, if one considers these six references in terms of their acceptability as 'best' evidence, only one article is a report of an experimental study whilst a further three papers report other non-experimental research findings.

The AMED search resulted in a total of 202 hits. Of these references 14 appeared to be relevant to the topic. Of the apparently relevant articles there were no duplications between the two AMED searches, indicating the value of using a variety of key words and searches within any one database. In terms of the hierarchy of evidence, only three of the identified articles appeared to be RCTs or experimental research and one was a meta-analysis. The remaining citations either gave no methodological information or were for qualitative research, surveys or case studies. Of the 14 identified articles, none were directly related to all aspects of the original evidence-based question. The majority were concerned with exercise or leisure rehabilitation, particularly with patients who had experienced strokes or cardiac problems with related depression.

One of the problems with this search is that one of the key terms, 'activity', is a very vague term which has a variety of meanings as was shown by the ways the thesaurus broke the term down. The hits tended to focus on leisure activities rather than the more OT notion of therapeutic and purposeful activity which was the original focus of the question. More details of this search and its results can be found in Taylor (1999).

Search 2

Question and search terms

What is the evidence for the value of horticulture as a purposeful activity and means of improving self esteem and confidence in clients with eating disorders?

Problem	*Intervention*	*Outcome*
Eating disorders: • anorexia • bulimia	Horticulture	Improve self-esteem • increase confidence in self • increase confidence in abilities

Search terms:

eating disorders	horticulture horticulture therapy gardening rehabilitation

Choice of databases

The focus of this question is a therapeutic activity, horticulture. Therefore, the databases to be searched should include a wide range of OT and other therapy references. Horticulture is also a topic of interest beyond health care and references and information could be available in a wide range of areas. The databases chosen to search were:

AMED
World Wide Web

To search the Web you need what is known as a 'search engine'. Search engines are Internet sites which have an automated search device (known as a 'crawler'). Crawlers search the Internet and collect together Web pages. The crawler then creates an index and catalogue of all the collected pages. However, the evidence-based OT should be aware that *no* attempt is made to review or assess the quality of these Web pages. If it is on the Web it will be included in the index. When you access a search engine you can search the index by using key words, just as if you were searching a database. The search engine will produce a list of *all* the Web sites in its index which contain the key word(s). These are known as *hits* and are ranked (by the search engine) according to their relevance to the key word(s). Relevance is defined, by the search engine, in terms of factors such as location (i.e. is the word in the title, the abstract, the text) and frequency, which might not translate into relevance for your particular search. However, *be warned* that Web searches can produce millions of hits!

There are a number of techniques available for refining Web searching, for example:

- " " (quotation marks) can be used to make a number of words into a phrase rather than separate terms (e.g. "occupational therap" or "horticulture therap")
- + indicates that a word must be present in all hits (e.g. +horticulture +therapy)
- – indicates that a word should be excluded from all hits (e.g. therapy – physical could be used to exclude references to physical therapy/physiotherapy)
- * can be used to truncate words where a number of word endings are possible (e.g. therap* would access both therapy and therapist)

Most search engines also have advanced search options where you can use Boolean search operators (e.g. AND, NOT, OR).

A number of search engines and sites exist including:

www.altavista.com
www.yahoo.co.uk
www.excite.co.uk
www.webcrawler.com

AltaVista is commonly thought of as one of the best search engines as it has a large and comprehensive index. For this reason it was chosen for this search.

Search strategy: comparing AMED and World Wide Web

AMED

- The search terms chosen were:
  - horticulture
  - horticulture therapy
  - eating disorders.
- AMED's thesaurus was used to refine the search terms. This proved interesting as 'horticulture' and 'horticulture therapy' did not exist on the AMED listing. 'Gardening' was, therefore, chosen as an alternative search term, 'eating disorders' was exploded to include all related terms and areas, e.g. anorexia and bulimia.
- 'horticulture' was used as a natural language search term and produced three hits.
- 'gardening' and 'eating disorders' were searched using the Boolean operator AND and produced three hits.
- 'gardening' alone produced 20 hits.
- It was then decided to combine 'eating disorders' and 'rehabilitation' (also exploded) to see if any other relevant articles could be found and this search resulted in 30 hits.

World Wide Web

- This used AltaVista's simple search facility.
- Using the terms ' "horticulture therapy" and "eating disorders" ', the search produced 1 080 000 hits! Note that " " was used to

indicate that horticulture therapy and eating disorders should be treated as phrases rather than separate search terms.

- As a way of attempting to refine this vast number of hits into something manageable and useful, AltaVista's advanced search facility was used.
- The advanced search facility allows the use of Boolean operators and date limits for the search and for the search to be refined by excluding certain search terms.
- Using the advanced search, "horticulture therapy" AND "eating disorders" provided a more modest 37 hits.
- Information is displayed on pages containing 10 hits at a time, each item can be expanded to link with the particular Web site.

Outcomes of search

Altogether the AMED search resulted in 56 hits from the various search terms and combinations of eating disorders/gardening/horticulture/rehabilitation. Of the 56 hits, 13 had relevance for the question with only one of these being a duplication (between the horticulture and the gardening searches). None of the identified articles addressed all of the aspects of the original evidence-based question. Articles were either case studies using horticulture in various mental health settings or reviews or case studies of OT with patients with eating disorders. The value of the use of the thesaurus is indicated in this search by the greater number of hits and relevant articles in the 'gardening' search in comparison to the 'horticulture' search, gardening being the word identified in the thesaurus.

Of the 37 sites and Web pages identified in the Internet search only four had any relevance to the question. The Web is a vast resource. However, it tends to be disorganised and idiosyncratic. Although it can allow access to up-to-date information from around the world, it is often a matter of luck and serendipity whether relevant information is accessed. AltaVista is only one of a number of search engines and the researcher may benefit from attempting the same search using a variety of search engines.

The combination of AMED and the Web resulted in a number of potential sources of information about horticulture as a therapeutic medium. The lack of research evidence for the value of horticulture therapy and the lack of any references suggesting the use of horticulture with patients with eating disorders indicates that this is a potentially useful area for further research.

Search 3

Question and search terms

> *What is the evidence for the value of anxiety management as a means of improving function/occupational performance/immunity/quality of life in clients who are HIV positive or who have AIDS?*

Problem	*Intervention*	*Outcome*
Anxiety in clients with HIV/AIDS	Anxiety management	Improved function and occupational performance; improved immunity; improved quality of life

Search terms:

HIV	anxiety management	activities of daily living
AIDS	stress management	quality of life
anxiety	rehabilitation	immune response

Choice of databases

This question covers a broader perspective than the previous questions. Anxiety management, as an intervention, may be carried out by a number of health care professionals. Databases that cover a broad health care perspective should be used. The databases chosen for the search were:

CINAHL
AMED

This search provided a useful opportunity to compare these two databases, which may be thought of as covering similar areas of interest.

Search strategy: comparing CINAHL and AMED

CINAHL

- The search terms chosen were:
  - anxiety
  - anxiety management
  - HIV and AIDS
  - immun* – truncated to access immune, immunity, etc.
- It was decided to use the terms as natural language rather than via the thesaurus, as this had proved successful in Search 2.
- The various search terms were combined, using AND, with varying degrees of success:
  - anxiety management – 28 hits
  - anxiety AND HIV/AIDS – 159 hits
  - anxiety management AND HIV/AIDS – no hits
  - anxiety AND immun* – 285 hits
  - anxiety AND immun* AND HIV/AIDS – 103 hits.

AMED

- The AMED search used the same terms as the CINAHL search, with rather fewer hits:
  - anxiety management – 20 hits
  - anxiety AND HIV/AIDS – 15 hits
  - anxiety management AND HIV/AIDS – no hits
  - anxiety AND immun* – 20 hits
  - anxiety AND immun* AND HIV/AIDS – 6 hits.

Outcomes of search

The CINAHL search produced a huge number of hits, whereas the AMED search produced a much more manageable number. When the output from both searches was compared the CINAHL search gave eight potentially relevant articles and the AMED search gave 12 relevant articles. However, there were five duplicates between the searches. This indicates that the CINAHL search gave little extra information for this topic, thus implying that, for topics which cover allied health care perspectives, the evidence-based OT might be best advised to choose AMED as the database of choice rather than CINAHL.

Search 4

Question and search terms

What is the evidence for the value of energy conservation as a means of improving quality of life/occupational performance and decreasing levels of fatigue in clients who experience high levels of fatigue associated with chronic illnesses such as MS, AIDS, RA?

Problem	*Intervention*	*Alternative interventions*	*Outcome*
Fatigue associated with: • MS • HIV/AIDS • RA	Energy conservation	Individual or group session; length of course; handouts and/ or discussion; self-help	Improved quality of life; increased occupational performance; decreased fatigue

Search terms:

fatigue multiple sclerosis HIV AIDS rheumatoid arthritis	energy conservation rehabilitation	education groups	activities of daily living quality of life

Choice of databases

This question covers a wide area and has both a rehabilitation and medical focus. The databases searched should give access to both medical and allied health literature. The databases chosen for the search were:

PubMed
AMED

Search strategy: comparing PubMed and AMED

PubMed

- This used PubMed's advanced search facility.
- PubMed has a MeSH browser which allows the searcher to refine the key terms to be used in the search. From the relatively long list of key terms outlined above an initial search was carried out using the MeSH terms 'fatigue' and 'rehabilitation' and the Boolean operator AND. This search identified 77 hits
- A further search using 'activities of daily living' AND 'fatigue' gave 46 hits, most of which were duplications of the fatigue/rehabilitation search.
- Further searches were carried out using the terms:
  - multiple sclerosis
  - rheumatoid arthritis
  - HIV
  - AIDS

  paired with both 'fatigue' and 'activities of daily living'. These searches identified a further 240 references.
- PubMed also has the phrase 'see related articles' by each citation, this was accessed for a number of selected articles and produced 174 further hits.

AMED

- Following the successful strategy for the PubMed search, 'fatigue' and 'rehabilitation' were chosen as the search terms.
- When fatigue was reviewed using the thesaurus it was not an accepted term, alternative terms included:
  - fatigue mental
  - fatigue syndrome chronic
  - muscle fatigue.
- Ignoring the thesaurus, fatigue was used as a 'natural word'.
- 'fatigue AND rehabilitation' were searched and produced 63 hits. To ensure that references to the specific illnesses were not being

missed, fatigue was combined with:

- multiple sclerosis – 20 hits
- rheumatoid arthritis – 9 hits
- HIV/AIDS – 6 hits.

Outcomes of search

Of the 537 hits identified by the PubMed searches, only 34 proved to be usefully related to the question, and of those only a small number appeared to be research-based articles. The most useful search was the first, using the terms fatigue/rehabilitation. Many of the items found on this search reappeared on other searches. The lessons to be learnt from this search are to identify the key elements of the question and to use these as the terms for the search, and not to make the search too elaborate by adding new terms just for the sake of including all the possible key terms. If the first terms have been well chosen they should produce the best results.

The results of the AMED search gave 98 hits in total. Of these, 23 were relevant to the question. However, five of these articles appeared in at least two PubMed searches. The two most productive searches were 'fatigue AND rehabilitation' and 'fatigue AND multiple sclerosis'. The success of the various combinations of search terms indicates that, unlike in the PubMed search, the evidence-based OT should not always be satisfied with the results of the first search terms.

The PubMed search was successful using the MeSH terms. However, the AMED search was more productive when natural language was used. The lesson from this search indicates that there are occasions when the thesaurus should be ignored and natural language should be used as search terms.

Search 5

Question and search terms

What is the evidence for the value of memory aids as a means of decreasing confusion and improving memory function and occupational performance in clients with memory impairment as a result of brain injury?

Problem	*Intervention*	*Alternative interventions*	*Outcome*
Memory impairment following brain injury	Memory aids	Group or individual sessions; education or activity	Decrease in confusion; increase in memory function; increase in occupational performance

Search terms:

brain injury head injury memory	rehabilitation memory aids	education groups	activities of daily living

Choice of databases

As this question is being used as part of a systematic review, the main evidence should be from RCTs. However, memory dysfunction is a subject that will also be discussed in social science literature. Databases covering both RCTs and social science literature were chosen for this search:

ASSIA
Cochrane Library

Search strategy: comparing ASSIA and Cochrane Library

ASSIA

- As the CD-ROM version of ASSIA was not available to the author, a hand-search of ASSIA year-volume by year-volume was carried out.
- The key terms used were:
  - memory
  - head injury
  - brain damage/injury.
- 40 hits were identified.

Cochrane Library

- The Cochrane Library has both simple and advanced search facilities. This search was carried out using the advanced search facility.
- Prior to searching, the MeSH thesaurus was used to refine and identify the most effective search terms.
- The following terms were identified as the most relevant terms for this question:
  - head injury
  - memory
  - memory disorders
  - rehabilitation.
- When all of the search terms were combined, using the Boolean operator AND, the search produced one hit.
- When the various terms were paired, for example:
  - head injury AND rehabilitation
  - memory AND rehabilitation

  a further 69 hits were identified.
- All of the hits were located in the Cochrane Controlled Trials Register.

Outcomes of search

Hand searching is probably the most effective but also the most time-consuming form of searching. However, it does allow for a great deal of selectivity when identifying appropriate hits. The 40 hits were all deemed to be useful and appropriate to the question. Because ASSIA includes all types of article (review and research) and all types of research methodology, a wide range of studies were identified, a number of which appeared to be RCTs. There was only one duplication with the Cochrane Library search, indicating the rather limited coverage of OT-specific literature in the Cochrane Library.

The Cochrane Library search identified 70 potentially relevant clinical trials. The results of the first, combined search identified one highly pertinent RCT. The searcher could have been satisfied with that one piece of information. However, the various paired searches identified a further 10 articles which described RCTs and CCTs of relevance to the question. The moral of this search is: never be satisfied with the first result, further searches may locate even more useful information.

The two databases used in this search appear to have been well balanced and to have provided a varied selection of references with minimal overlap. This combination of databases indicates the value of using a variety of contrasting databases for any evidence-based search.

Review of the databases

Having given an overview of the various searches, it now seems appropriate to review the various databases used in these searches and to highlight key points to successful searching. All of the databases searched have their strengths and, as indicated above, should be used in combination to provide access to the widest range of evidence. It should be noted that the databases are listed, below, in alphabetical order and not in order of preference or perceived value. Table 2.1 summarises the key aspects of each of the databases used in these searches. Further, more detailed, information on these databases, together with other sources of evidence, can be found in Chapter 7.

- **AMED**
  AMED is probably the best resource for OT intervention and general health care literature (especially in comparison to CINAHL, see Search 4). Natural language should be used as search terms in initial searches and, only when this is unsuccessful should the thesaurus be used. However, AMED's indexing is not always very thorough and searches may provide fewer hits than expected due to the limitations of the indexing rather than due to lack of published literature. If, for example, you use 'systematic review' as your key words (see Chapter 4) you will access literature reviews as well as *systematic* reviews.

Table 2.1 Summary of databases.

Database	Coverage	Relevance to occupational therapy*	Rigour of content	Access	Effort required
AMED	Main focus is therapies and rehabilitation	Very relevant	Mixed – must be critically appraised	Should be accessible through health care (academic and hospital) libraries	Some training advisable for most efficient use
ASSIA	Focus on social sciences and social aspects of care	Fairly relevant, but highly relevant for some topics	Mixed – must be critically appraised	Should be accessible through academic libraries, may be accessible through health or social care libraries	Some training advisable for most efficient use
CINAHL	Main focus is nursing with some rehabilitation literature	Fairly relevant	Mixed – must be critically appraised	Should be accessible through health care (academic and hospital) libraries	Some training advisable for most efficient use
Cochrane Library	Main focus is RCTs and systematic reviews	Highly relevant for some topics, otherwise of some relevance	High-quality and rigorous information	Should be accessible through health care (academic and hospital) libraries.	Straightforward; however, some training advisable for most efficient use

OTDBASE	OT specific literature	Highly relevant	Mixed – must be critically appraised	On the Internet, by subscription	Straightforward and easy to use
PubMed/MEDLINE	Medical focus, although a broad definition of medicine	Fairly relevant	Mixed – must be critically appraised	PubMed is available free on the Internet. MEDLINE should be accessible through health care (academic and hospital) libraries	Some training advisable for most efficient use
World Wide Web	Anything and everything!	Limited relevance, but it will depend on the topic	Unknown – needs very careful appraisal	Internet access required.	Straightforward; however, some training advisable for most efficient use

* Relevance to OT is defined in a scale from:
very relevant
highly relevant
fairly relevant
some relevance
limited relevance

- **ASSIA**
  ASSIA contains a breadth of social science literature and might be a useful second source of evidence in combination with AMED/ Cochrane, etc.
- **CINAHL**
  CINAHL performed less well in comparison to AMED. However, CINAHL would be a useful source if the question demanded a greater emphasis on nursing literature.
- **Cochrane Library**
  The Cochrane Library is easy to use and has a good help section, which can be used in conjunction with the Guide (McKinnell & Elliott, 1997). It is probably the best source for RCTs and controlled clinical trials (CCTs), especially in medicine, but is getting better in its inclusion of OT and OT-related literature.
- **OTDBASE**
  OTDBASE does the key word choosing for you. This might be useful for the novice searcher. However, it does not allow for very specific or sophisticated searches.
- **PubMed**
  PubMed is an excellent resource for medical literature, but searches can produce overwhelming numbers of hits. The advanced search facility is very useful. Unlike AMED, PubMed searches should begin with the MeSH thesaurus and only once this is exhausted should natural language be used.
- **World Wide Web**
  The World Wide Web is a vast resource. However, no attempt has been made to organise information on the Web and any search of the Web will generate a large number of irrelevant hits and, quite probably, a great deal of frustration.

See Chapter 7 for information on other databases and sources of information/evidence such as:

- OMNI
- *Bandolier*

- *Effective Health Care Bulletin*
- *Evidence-based Medicine/Mental Health/Nursing* etc.

Pointers for successful searching include:

- Use more than one resource/database
- Be creative with the key words, and combinations of terms
- Any search will be limited by the effectiveness of the indexing in any database
- Any search is only as good as the original question
- Use the thesaurus, but trust natural language first, especially with AMED
- Use the advanced search, where possible, to combine terms
- Allow plenty of time
- Search with a 'buddy' (a colleague or friend), two heads will produce more refined search terms and may provide a more critical evaluation of the usefulness of any hit
- Decide whether to display *brief fields* or *all fields* as the search result; all fields will give the abstract but can produce extremely lengthy search results if the citation includes references as well as an abstract

Activity

- Refine the question you developed at the end of Chapter 1, identify the key terms and add terms to those you have previously identified
- Identify your data/information source, which library will you use?
- Work out your budget of time and money available to answer your question
- Identify possible sources of help with the search, e.g. librarians, students
- Identify the database(s) that will be most useful for your search
- Develop your search strategy:
  - Refine your search terms
  - Identify the limits to the search:
    - language of article
    - year of publication
    - specific journals
    - research articles only
- Carry out a search

Accessing evidence

Having completed your search and found a number of useful looking references, the next task for the evidence-based OT is to locate the relevant articles. This is not always a simple task. Databases allow access to literature from around the world. However, libraries (even the best-stocked libraries) rarely have copies of every journal you might need. Any library, however small and given time, should be able to obtain most documents for you as all libraries are part of a network of public, health care or academic libraries nation-wide.

If the journal you require is held by the library, you can read the article before deciding if the article really is of relevance to your search and worth photocopying. If the library does not hold the journal you require, they will be able to order a copy of any article either from other libraries in the region or from the British Library, through the Inter-Library Loan scheme. It is also sometimes possible to download copies of articles or documents from databases or the Internet. The thing to remember with any of these methods of accessing articles is that there is a cost involved. Photocopying must be paid for and Inter-Library Loans are usually accompanied by a fee. Therefore, be selective about which references are particularly relevant to your question, otherwise you could be spending a great deal of time and money accessing information that is interesting but not directly relevant to your question.

Possibly the most important resource for any evidence-based OT is the local librarian. Librarians are experts in dealing with information. They can carry out searches for you or they can help you to carry out your own search. Once the search is completed the librarian can help the evidence-based OT to access the articles, books and documents that are required. Most libraries will offer a programme of tutorials and help-sessions on:

- Introduction to the library services
- Basic and more advanced searching on a range of databases
- Managing references and developing your own database

Librarians are invaluable sources of knowledge and help. Make friends with your local librarian.

A word about copyright. Copyright is complex and is governed by law. The copyright laws limit the amount of material that can be copied from any published work without the permission of the copyright owner. Infringement of the copyright can lead to prosecution. Copies made by the individual who will be using the material must be for the purposes of research or private study and must not constitute a 'substantial' part of the work. This is interpreted as:

- One article from any one issue of a journal
- One chapter from a book

Activity

- Get to know your local librarian, describe your areas of interest and ask to be kept up to date with information relevant to your areas of interest
- Review the budget you developed above to include the cost of photocopying and Inter-Library Loans

Storing and indexing evidence

Having completed the search and acquired all of the relevant material, two tasks remain. The value of the evidence must be appraised, this will be discussed in Chapter 3–5, and the references and material must be organised and stored.

There are three possible options for organising evidence:

- Using folders, files or a filing cabinet to store references, articles and notes
- Using a card index system for references and notes
- Using a personal database to store references and notes

The only one of these which may be unfamiliar to the reader is probably the personal database approach.

The personal database approach allows you to store references and notes on computer and thus facilitates the creation of reports by allowing material to be copied from the database and incorporated into the report text. Two types of database software are available:

- General databases, such as Access;
- Specialist personal bibliographic software (PBS), such as EndNote

The advantage of PBS software is that it is designed specifically to handle bibliographic information. The disadvantage is the cost of this specialist software. Most personal computers will have some form of pre-loaded database program included as part of the sales package. General database programs, such as Access, usually have pre-existing templates which may include a bibliographic database template. This will make creating an evidence-based database somewhat simpler.

Whatever method of organisation you choose, you should ensure that the following information is included:

- Full bibliographic citation
- Appraisal notes and comments
- Useful quotations, including page reference
- Location of hard copy of article
- Source of original reference

Activity

- Identify what database software (specialised and general) is available for your use
- Identify sources of help available to assist your use of the database software
- Design an organisation and storage system

Further reading/resources

The following further reading and resources will allow the reader to develop a greater knowledge of the various resources available to aid evidence-based OTs in their search for useful and relevant evidence to underpin their practice.

Bandolier

Chartered Society of Physiotherapy (1996) *Literature Searching: Where to Go and What to Look For.* London: Chartered Society of Physiotherapy.

Dale, P. (ed.) (1997) *Guide to Libraries and Information Sources in Medicine and Health Care.* London: The British Library.

Effective Health Care Bulletin

Evidence Based Healthcare: A Resource Pack – http://drsdesk.sghms.ac.uk/Starnet/pack.htm

Greenhalgh, T. (1997) *How to Read a Paper*. London: BMJ Publishing Group.

Greyson, L. (1997) *Evidence-based Medicine: An Overview and Guide to the Literature*. London: The British Library.

Introduction to Information Mastery – http://www.familypractice.msu.ed/InfoMastery/

McKinnell, I. & Elliott, J. (1997) *The Cochrane Library: Self-Training Guide and Notes.* Oxford: Anglia & Oxford NHS Executive. http://www.lib.jr2.ox.ac.uk/nhserdd/aordd/evidence/clibtrng.htm

Reed, K.L. & Cunningham, S. (1997) *Internet Guide for Rehabilitation Professionals.* Philadelphia: JB Lippincott Co.

ScHARR – Finding the evidence – http://www.shef.ac.uk/~scharr/finding.html

Reynard, K.W. & Reynard, J.M.E. (eds) (1996) *ASLIB Directory of Information Sources in the United Kingdom.* London: ASLIB.

ScHARR – Netting the evidence – http://www.shef.ac.uk/~scharr/ir/netting.html

ScHARR – Trawling the Net – http://www.shef.ac.uk/~scharr/ir/trawling.html

The Clinician's Lament: How do I keep up with the literature? – http://www.nyam.org/library/ebm/index.htm

User Guides to the Medical Literature – http://hiru.hirunet.mcmaster.ca/ebm/userguid/default.htm

York Centre for Reviews and Dissemination – guidelines for developing complex searches: http://www.york.ac.uk/inst/crd/report4#appendix1

Chapter 3
USING CLINICAL TRIALS AS EVIDENCE

It has often been said that randomised controlled trials (RCTs) and controlled clinical trials (CCTs) are not methods used frequently in OT research (Taylor, 1997). However, this is beginning to change. An OT RCT has recently been published in the prestigious *Journal of the American Medical Association* (JAMA) (Clark *et al.* 1997). A preparatory search for this chapter revealed 78 RCTs and CCTs listed in the Cochrane Controlled Trials Register when 'occupational therapy' was used as the search term. A search of AMED using the terms:

random* (truncated because of the different spellings of randomised)
control* (again truncated because the terms randomised controlled and randomised control trial are both used)
trial
AND
occupational therapy

revealed eight RCTs, of which only one was duplicated in the Cochrane search. Examples of OT RCTs include: Liddle *et al.* (1996), Przybylski *et al.* (1996), Zisselman *et al.* (1996), Baker *et al.* (1997) and Logan *et al.* (1997).

Randomised controlled trials are seen as the gold standard for evidence. Therefore it is important for evidence-based OTs to be able to understand and appraise RCTs and CCTs. This chapter will draw on examples of published OT RCTs and CCTs to outline the nature of clinical trials (these are presented in the boxes within the text). The findings of these trials will then be outlined and used as illustrations to explain the statistical analysis used in RCTs. It is not the intention of this chapter to make the reader a competent data analyst but to enable the reader to read and understand the results section of any research paper, rather than skip over the results and move straight to the discussion. Chapter 7 includes an annotated bibliography which will highlight possible sources of further information on research design and analysis.

What are clinical trials?

The aim of any clinical trial is to test the effectiveness of an intervention, whether in comparison to no intervention or in comparison to another form of intervention. The most rigorous form of clinical trial is the randomised controlled trial (RCT). An alternative, and less rigorous, form of clinical trial is the controlled clinical trial (CCT).

Randomised controlled trials (RCTs)

The reason RCTs are seen as such useful sources of evidence for assessing the effectiveness of any intervention is because of the process of randomisation. This means that, having decided who the sample population is to be and setting clear parameters for who is acceptable to the trial, each participant has an equal likelihood of being allocated to the intervention group or to the control (non-intervention) group. This ensures that any bias is minimised and that the two groups of participants are as similar as possible. Without random allocation of participants, the researcher might choose the 'best' clients to be members of the intervention group. If the participants in the two groups are as similar as possible the researcher can, then, state with confidence that any differences at the end of the study are due to the intervention and not to differences between the groups.

Box 3.1

The study of Logan *et al.* (1997) compared the effect of an enhanced Social Services intervention with the normal Social Services intervention for a group of stroke patients. On discharge from hospital stroke patients were referred to the local Social Services department. The referrals were then randomly allocated to the normal or the enhanced service. The enhanced service consisted of an OT whose sole remit was to work with stroke clients. This meant that her referrals were seen more quickly and her remit also included home therapy as well as the provision of equipment. Participants were assessed, using functional and psychological measures, at 3 months and 6 months following referral.

Any RCT will consist of a number of phases, as illustrated in Fig. 3.1.

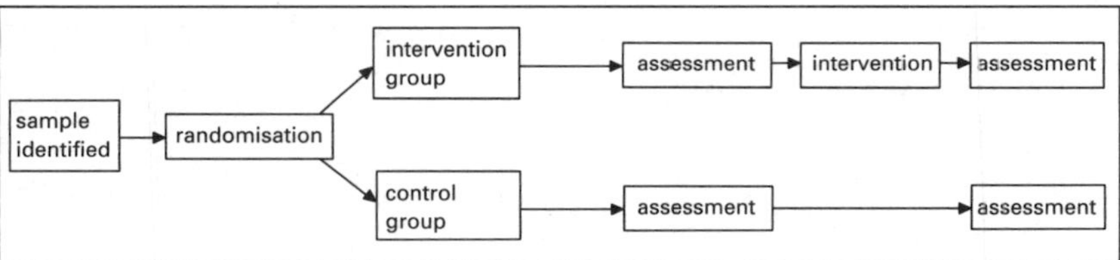

Fig. 3.1 Phases of a random controlled trial (RCT).

Box 3:2

The study of Clark *et al.* (1997) attempted to explore the role of OT in health promotion by evaluating the effectiveness of a preventative OT intervention for older adults living independently in the community. Participants were randomly allocated to one of three groups: an OT group, a social activity group or a non-intervention group. Both the social activity and the non-intervention groups were seen as control groups. Participants were assessed at the start of the study and again at the end of the 9-month study period on a range of self-administered questionnaires measuring physical and social function, health, life satisfaction and depressive symptoms.

The control group may receive no intervention, as in the Liddle *et al.* (1996) study, the existing intervention, as in the Logan *et al.* (1997) and Przybylski *et al.* (1996) studies, an alternative intervention as in the Baker *et al.* (1997) and Zisselman *et al.* (1996) studies, or a combination as in the Clark *et al.* (1997) study.

Box 3.3

In a study of the short-term and long-term effects of a Snoezelen environment on older people with dementia, Baker *et al.* (1997) randomly assigned patients to a series of eight activity sessions of Snoezelen sessions. Assessment took place pre-trial, mid-trial, post-trial and after an (unspecified) follow-up period. Measures of behaviour, mood and cognition were used.

The reason for using an alternative or existing intervention, rather than no intervention, reduces the risks of any placebo effect. The control group provides a baseline against which any changes in the intervention group can be compared to assess whether the intervention has been effective.

Box 3.4

Zisselman *et al.* (1996) used an RCT to evaluate the effects of pet therapy on older adults on an in-patient psychiatric unit. The intervention group had a 1-hour interaction with a dog everyday for a 5-day period, whilst the control group spent the hour in an exercise group. Assessment before and after the intervention period consisted of a standardised observation of self-care, orientation, mood and behaviour.

Controlled clinical trials (CCTs)

Controlled clinical trials also aim to assess the effectiveness of an intervention by comparing two groups of participants. However, for practical or ethical reasons in these trials, it has not been possible to randomly allocate participants to the respective groups. Controlled clinical trials often use pre-existing divisions as a way of dividing participants into intervention and control groups, e.g. by using participants from different geographical areas or patients on different wards.

Box 3.5

Sanford *et al.* (1996) used a CCT to assess the effectiveness of an interactive computer and video instruction package to teach OT and physiotherapy students about arthritis. The study took place over 2 academic years. In the first year of the study students were taught using traditional classroom methods. In the second year of the study the interactive package replaced the traditional teaching methods.

The phases of a CCT are the same as those of a RCT, in terms of assessment, intervention and re-assessment. The problem with any CCT is that the two groups cannot be assumed to be as similar as they would be if randomisation had taken place. Any research papers should be appraised carefully to ensure that the groups being compared are similar on all key variables.

Box 3.6

In a study evaluating OT intervention in maintaining the independence and quality of life of older people, Liddle *et al.* (1996) randomly allocated participants who had been assessed by an OT as needing equipment/home modifications/services to an intervention or non-intervention group. The intervention group were given the equipment, etc., that had been recommended. The non-intervention group did not have the OT's recommendations carried out. Clients who were assessed to require no further intervention formed a further control group. Assessment measures included quality of life and functional activity. Participants were reviewed 6 months after the initial interview.

Box 3.7

In a study covering a 2-year period, Przybylski *et al.* (1996) assessed the value of increasing the ratio of OTs and physiotherapists (PTs) to patients in a nursing home setting. Residents in a nursing home were randomly allocated to an enhanced OT/PT group, where the ratio was 1.0 FTE (full-time equivalent) PT and 1.0 FTE OT per 50 residents or to a control group, where the ratio was 1.0 FTE PT and 1.0 FTE OT per 200 residents. Functional independence was measured at 6-month intervals over a 2-year period.

Both RCTs and CCTs are invaluable methods for assessing the effectiveness of a particular intervention with a clearly defined client group or population. Both research methods require rigorous standardisation of procedures and measures, which will result in objective and statistical analysis of the intervention outcomes. As we have seen, these methods are becoming more frequently used in OT research. However, the more subjective elements are ignored by RCTs and CCTs. Both RCTs and CCTs will not provide evidence of how the client perceived the intervention or anything about the client's experience of, or satisfaction with, the intervention. They will, however, be able to answer the question 'did the intervention work?' These methods of research will not be able to answer the questions 'how was it for the client?' nor 'was the client satisfied with the intervention process and outcome?' Only qualitative research methods, which are discussed in Chapter 5, can answer these types of questions.

The magic *P*-value – an outline of probability and statistical analysis, relevant to appraising RCT evidence

When reading a research paper the part most people dread, and therefore skip over or ignore, is the results section. This section is always full of numbers and symbols which often make little sense to readers unless they have a sound grasp of statistical concepts. The aim of this part of the chapter is to help you to feel more confident when reading the results section of a RCT report and especially to focus on the key pieces of information needed to appraise a RCT.

Statistical analysis can be divided into two groups. Each group of analysis serves a different function. The first type of analysis is *descriptive analysis*. This allows the researcher to describe the data and to make general observations about the data and the findings. The second type of analysis is *inferential analysis*. This is where the various participant groups' results are compared, differences between groups are assessed and conclusions are drawn. The main task of inferential analysis is to assess the likelihood of any differences between the groups having occurred by chance. This is referred to as *probability* and is expressed as a *P*-value.

Descriptive analysis

One way of describing a participant group is to use *percentages* as a way of indicating what proportion of the group represent different variables or characteristics, e.g. age, gender, ethnicity, diagnosis, social class. In the study by Logan *et al.* (1997), 57% of the participants were male, 45% had left hemisphere damage and 15% had dysphasia.

Another method of describing a population is to use the average or *mean*. The mean age of participants in the enhanced group of the study by Przybylski *et al.* (1996) was 83 years and of the control group was 86 years (see Box 3.8). The statistical symbol for the mean is $\bar{x}$. The mean, however, only gives a single figure, which describes a middle point in the data. The mean does not give any idea of the overall spread, dispersion or variation of the data. The *range* and the *standard deviation* (SD) give the reader information about the spread and the distribution of scores. The range is denoted by the lowest and the highest scores. The standard deviation is a method of describing the spread of scores and how close to the mean the majority (68%) of the scores lie. The larger the standard deviation the greater the spread of scores. Together the mean, range and standard deviation give the reader a clearer overview of the data being presented.

Box 3.8

In the study of Przybylski *et al.* (1996) the mean age of the enhanced group was 83 years but for the control group the mean age was 86 years, which might imply that the control group were older than the enhanced group. However, the range of ages for the enhanced group was 62–97 years and for the control group it was 63–101 years. The mean age of the control group might have been influenced by one or two 101-year-olds. These two descriptors together give the reader more information with which to judge the validity of the results.

The study of Logan *et al.* (1997) into Social Services OT showed the mean age of the enhanced group was 71 with a standard deviation of 10.2 whilst the mean age of the control group was 74 with a standard deviation of 11.5. This means that 68% of the enhanced group were aged 71 ± 10.2, i.e. between 60.8 and 81.2, whilst 68% of the control group were aged between 62.5 and 85.5 (74 ± 11.5). From these figures it might be assumed that the control group was somewhat older than the enhanced group.

However, statistical analysis of the ages of participants in both the Przybylski *et al.* and the Logan *et al.* studies showed that the enhanced and control groups were not significantly different.

As the mean can be affected by extreme values, other methods of describing the mid-points or *central tendency* of the data are also used, especially where the data may include extreme values. The most commonly used alternative measure of central tendency is the *median*. This is the actual mid-point if the data were set out in order. Where the data are expressed as a number of categories, e.g. age bands, social class, professional groups, then the *mode* is used to describe the category most frequently recorded.

Box 3.9

Because the length of stay in hospital following a cardiovascular accident (CVA) can vary between a few days to many months, Logan *et al.* (1997) used the median rather than the mean to describe the length-of-stay data in their study. The median and range of length of time in hospital for the control group was 45 days, ranging from 4 to 238 days. For the enhanced group the median was 39 days and the range was from 6 to 252 days.

Descriptive analysis can be written in the text of the results, presented in table format e.g. participant characteristics and demographic information, or displayed in graph or chart form, e.g. Baker *et al.* (1997).

Inferential statistics

As mentioned above, the aim of inferential statistics is to compare data from the intervention group and the control group and to determine whether any differences in outcome between these groups would have occurred by chance. In other words, whether the researcher can be certain that the improvement (or change) in the intervention group was due to the intervention or was due to chance factors. How confident researchers can be in the effectiveness of their intervention is referred to as the *level of significance* of the findings. This is expressed in terms of the *P*-value. *P* stands for probability.

The probability, or likelihood, that any difference between intervention and control groups can be anything between 1.0000 and 0.0000. The smaller the value of *P*, the more confident the researcher can be that any differences are not due to chance factors. Whether the differences are seen and accepted as due to chance factors is not, however, left to an arbitrary decision by the researcher. Research convention tends to accept 0.05 as the cut-off point. Above 0.05 and results are described as *not significant* (NS), in other words the differences between the groups must be seen as due to chance factors. Below 0.05 and the results are described as *significant*, or statistically significant, and the differences are accepted as not being due to chance factors. What a probability value of 0.05 means is that if the study were to be repeated 100 times, in 95 of the studies you would get the same result.

Accepting a level of probability as acceptable is all about risk and the level of risk the researcher, and the reader, is prepared to accept when considering whether the results of the study are an error. Figure 3.2 illustrates how probability and risk are related.

The researcher should state in the results section what level of significance is being accepted. Liddle *et al.* (1996: 576) by saying, 'there was no difference at the level of significance 0.01' were indicating that they accepted 0.01 (1 in 100) as their cut-off point. Clark *et al.* (1997) and Logan *et al.* (1997) indicated that 0.05 (1 in 20) was acceptable and Przybylski *et al.* (1996) were prepared to

If a study were repeated, how likely is it that **NO** differences would be found or that any differences between the intervention and control groups would be due to chance factors?

1.0000 ———————————————— 0.0000

very likely — very unlikely

P-value	Likelihood	Ratio
0.80	Very likely	4 in 5
0.50	Pretty likely	1 in 2
0.05	Fairly unlikely	1 in 20
0.01	Pretty unlikely	1 in 100
0.001	Very unlikely	1 in 1000

Fig. 3.2 An overview of probability and risk.

accept values as high as 0.08 (8 in 100). Pereira-Maxwell (1998) proposed that to allow interpretation and appraisal of research, the exact *P*-value should be stated rather than NS (for non-significant results) or $P < 0.05$ (for significant results).

The process of determining the *P*-value of any data is through a *statistical test*. The statistical test will allow a numerical value to be calculated from which the *P*-value can be determined. The types of statistical test are many and various, and include:

- t tests
- χ^2 tests (chi squared)
- Mann–Whitney U-tests
- ANOVA

The type of test used will depend on a number of factors, including the number of participants in each group and the type of data. Any researcher should explain what tests were chosen and the reasoning behind the choice. Further details of statistical analysis can be found in any research or statistics text (e.g. Munro and Page (1993)). Although the results section of any report will contain a wealth of information, the important aspect for any evidence-based OT to focus on is the *P*-value.

Statistical significance will allow the researcher to accept or reject an intervention or to argue that an intervention might be effective in improving certain outcomes for a particular client group. Thus Przybylski *et al.* (1996: 554) were able to conclude that

> 'increasing the amount of PT/OT can have a positive effect on the functional status ... of long-term care residents.'

However, this gives little indication of the *clinical significance* of the results in terms of the size of the treatment effect. It does not answer the question 'if I use this intervention, how many patients will I need to treat before I see one improvement?' or 'which patients will benefit most from this intervention?' or 'how much money will this intervention save/cost me?' A result may be statistically significant but be too small to be of value in terms of treatment. Clinical significance and the effectiveness of interventions can be assessed by measures such as confidence intervals (CIs), numbers needed to treat (NNT), odds ratios (ORs) and relative risk.

Measures of clinical significance

Confidence intervals (CI) are ways of estimating where the 'true' result for any population lies. The findings of a study may give results in terms of, for example, a mean improvement score. The confidence interval will allow you to judge the strength of that result in terms of the upper and lower values that are potentially possible for the given result. Confidence intervals are expressed as a percentage, with 95% being the most commonly used. The narrower the distance, or interval, between the values the more confident you can be in the result.

Box 3.10

Liddle *et al.* (1996) compared the percentage of people in the intervention group and the control group who had maintained satisfactory levels of outcomes. The confidence intervals for each figure were also recorded. Thus in the intervention group 64% of participants maintained a satisfactory score on the Life Satisfaction Index. The 95%CI for this figure was 50–78. In other words, the 'true' result could be anything from 50 to 78% of participants maintaining a satisfactory Life Satisfaction Index score.

Liddle *et al.* (1996) also expressed their findings in terms of *relative risk*. This is a measure of assessing the 'risk' or likelihood of a given event for one group of participants in comparison to another group (Pereira-Maxwell, 1998). If there is no difference in risk between the groups the relative risk value is 1. If the risk or likelihood is lower for the intervention group the value is less than 1 and greater than 1 if the risk is higher.

Box 3.11

Liddle *et al.* (1996) used relative risk to assess whether the intervention group would maintain satisfactory outcome levels. For the Life Satisfaction Index the relative risk was 0.9 with a 95%CI of 0.7–1.3. This can be interpreted as expecting the intervention group to do slightly less well in comparison to the control group in terms of maintaining satisfactory outcomes on the Life Satisfaction Index scale. However, the CI indicates that the intervention group might do better than the control group.

Numbers needed to treat (NNT) is a way of measuring the impact of an intervention in terms of how many people need to be treated in order to prevent one negative outcome (Pereira-Maxwell, 1998). In other words, a NNT of 25 would mean that for every 25 patients treated one patient would avoid the negative or adverse effect. Sackett *et al.* (1997) cited the example of intensive insulin therapy as a means of preventing neuropathy in diabetic patients. The evidence suggests a NNT of 15, which would mean for every 15 diabetic patients treated with an intensive insulin regime one patient would be prevented from developing diabetic neuropathy. Thus, the smaller the NNT the more effective the intervention.

A final measure of clinical significance is the *odds ratio* (OR). This measure is more commonly seen in systematic reviews and meta-analyses. Chapter 4 discusses systematic reviews and will include an explanation of odds ratios.

Before we consider how to appraise a RCT as a source of evidence, it is worth noting the effect that publication bias might have on the availability of RCT evidence (Gray, 1997). Some journals will only publish research where the results have achieved a 0.05 level of statistical significance. This means that research where the findings are not significant will not be published. This could mean that valuable evidence of the ineffectiveness of interventions is not published. In terms of the research discussed in this chapter, only the Przybylski *et al.* (1996), Baker *et al.* (1997), Clark *et al.* (1997) and Logan *et al.* (1997) studies found significant effects for the various forms of OT intervention under investigation. The Liddle *et al.* (1996) and Zisselman *et al.* (1996) studies found no significant differences between their intervention and control groups. However Sanford *et al.* (1996) found mixed significant and non-significant results for the effectiveness of the various teaching methods used in their CCT.

Appraising clinical trials

The focus of this chapter, and the following chapters on systematic reviews and qualitative research, is to provide the evidence-based OT with the skills needed to be able to critically appraise research evidence. However, this focus on critical appraisal begs two questions:

- What is critical appraisal?
- Why is critical appraisal of research evidence necessary?

Critical appraisal allows the evidence-based OT the opportunity to assess the value and trustworthiness of a piece of research within the context of practice and within a structured framework. The structure of the critical appraisal process allows the evidence-based OT to review not just the findings of the research but the whole research process. It is, however, important to bear in mind that no research or research paper is without its flaws. Critical appraisal does not mean taking a research paper apart and spitting out the bits! The flaws of the research should be weighed and evaluated carefully but should be viewed in the context of whether the flaws make you question the conclusions of the researchers. Critical appraisal should be positive rather than negative. Research should be read with an open mind and the ability to challenge your own, as well as the researcher's, ideas and assumptions.

Using a critical appraisal approach to reading research literature will encourage the evidence-based OT not to ignore, or skip over, the 'complicated' (results) sections of a research paper. Skipping over parts of an article may lead to misinterpretation of findings or accepting (or rejecting) the author's conclusions based on an inaccurate, or incorrect, interpretation of the research. Critical appraisal is often more interesting if it is not a solitary activity, so that the findings and ideas can be discussed and ideas and comments can be challenged and reviewed. Chapter 6 will discuss how journal clubs can be used as a way of sharing critical appraisals of research literature.

The appraisal of any article should address three broad areas:

- Are the results valid?
- What are the results?
- How will these results help me work with my clients?

The first area asks questions which will help you to appraise the rigour of the research and to ask the question 'is this good research?' The second area will ask questions which help you to assess the significance, both statistical and clinical, of the results. The final area enables you to reflect on whether the findings of the research have any direct relation or impact on your areas of OT practice. Table 3.1 gives an overview of the questions to ask when appraising a RCT. These questions are based on the questions developed as part of the Critical Appraisal Skills Programme (CASP) initiative with some additions, which the author felt were relevant to evidence-based OT (see Chapter 7 for more information about the CASP initiative).

Table 3.1 Questions to ask when critically appraising a clinical trial.

Are the results valid?

- Did the trial address a clearly focused issue?
- Was the assignment of participants to treatments randomised?
- Were all the participants who entered the trial properly accounted for at its conclusion?
- Is the literature review appropriate?
- Were participants, health workers and study personnel 'blind' to the treatment?
- Were the groups similar at the start of the trial?
- Apart from the experimental intervention, were the groups treated equally?
- Were ethical issues considered?

What are the results?

- Was there an adequate description of the data collection methods used?
- Were the methods of analysis appropriate, clearly described and justified?
- What are the key findings?
- How significant were the results?

How will the results help me work with my clients?

- Can the results be applied to the local population of my practice and clients?
- Were all the important outcomes considered?
- Are the benefits of the intervention worth the harms and the costs?

The use of a checklist, or series of questions, as a useful tool for critically appraising literature has been advocated by a number of authors, including Gray (1997), Greenhalgh (1997) and Sackett *et al*. (1997). The various questions will now be expanded. Table 3.2 gives a worked example of a critical appraisal of a RCT (Logan *et al*. 1997).

Table 3.2 Worked example of a critical appraisal of a randomised controlled trial (RCT) using: Logan, P.A., Ahern, J., Gladman, J.R. & Lincoln, N.B. (1997) A randomized controlled trial of enhanced Social Services occupational therapy for stroke patients. *Clinical Rehabilitation*, **11**(2), 107–13.

Question	Yes/no/ can't tell	Comments
Are the results valid?		
Did the trial address a clearly focused issue?	Yes	The research had a clear objective: To determine whether stroke patients referred to the Social Services OT service would benefit from an enhanced service, in comparison to the usual service. The population is clearly stated: Stroke patients, discharged from hospital and referred to the OT service. Outcomes and outcome measures were clearly defined: The focus was on functional improvement as measured by the Nottingham Extended ADL Scale (EADL), the Barthel Index, the General Health Questionnaire (GHQ) and a tally of the number of pieces of equipment issued. However, it was assumed that the reader was familiar with these measures and so no detail was given about the measures.
Was the assignment of participants to treatments randomised?	Yes	Following referral to the OT service, participants were randomly allocated to the intervention group or the control group by the OT administrator. Following randomisation, formal consent to be involved in the study was gained.

Contd

Table 3.2 *Contd.*

Question	Yes/no/ can't tell	Comments
Were all the participants who entered the trial properly accounted for at its conclusion?	Yes	Participants were seen at 3-month and 6-month follow-up and a table in the text gives a full account of all participants. The drop-out rates were not significantly different for the two groups.
If the answers to these screening questions are 'Yes' is it worth carrying on with the appraisal?	Yes	Proceed with the detailed appraisal.
Is the literature review appropriate?	Yes	Although the Introduction is brief, it does provide an adequate background to the study and its context.
Were participants, health workers and study personnel 'blind' to the treatment?	Can't tell	It is not stated whether the participants were aware of which group they had been allocated to. The two study groups were seen and treated by different therapists, and so they would, probably, be aware of which group their clients were in. The outcome measures were completed by an independent assessor who was blind to the treatment groups.
Were the groups similar at the start of the trial?	Yes	A table in the text outlines the comparisons between the two participant groups. They were compared by: • Age • Sex • % living alone • % who experienced dysphasia • % of participants with left hemisphere damage • Median days in hospital. There were no significant differences between the groups on any of these measures.

Contd

Table 3.2 *Contd.*

Question	Yes/no/ can't tell	Comments
		However, no baseline data of activities of daily living (ADL) function (i.e. using any of the study outcome measures) was given. Therefore, it was impossible to assess whether the groups were functionally similar at the start of the study.
Apart from the experimental intervention, were the groups treated equally?	Yes	The intervention group received more therapy, in a quicker time frame, but this was the nature of the study as not only outcomes but also the nature of therapy will be influenced by the use of an enhanced OT service.
Were ethical issues considered?	Can't tell	The issue of consent was discussed. However, other ethical issues such as confidentiality, distress, etc., were not discussed. The control group was not being denied intervention and the OT service was involved in its usual routine manner.
What are the results?		
Was there an adequate description of the data collection methods used?	Yes	The outcome measures used (see above) were standardised, commonly used, assessments. A clear overview of the data collection process was given.
Were the methods of analysis appropriate, clearly described and justified?	Yes/ can't tell	Although the analysis is appropriate, no attempt is made to outline why particular methods of analysis were chosen.
What are the key findings?	—	A table provides a clear overview of the differences in therapy given to the two groups. A table provides a clear overview comparing the various outcome measures between the two groups.

Contd

Table 3.2 *Contd.*

Question	Yes/no/ can't tell	Comments
		A final table compares the equipment and adaptations provided for the two groups. The results appear to provide clear answers to the research questions.
How significant were the results?	—	In terms of the comparison of therapy, the significant differences were: • Speed of 1st visit ($P<0.01$) • Number of visits ($P<0.01$) • Amount of therapy ($P<0.01$) In terms of the functional outcome measures, the significant differences were: • EADL at 3 months ($P<0.01$) • GHQ ($P<0.01$). Apart from the provision of stair rails ($P<0.01$) there were no significant differences in the number of pieces of equipment or adaptations provided for the two groups. Although there were some differences between the groups, especially at the 3-month follow-up, the differences are not large. However, there is some evidence to support the use of a dedicated stroke OT within a Social Services team.
How will the results help me work with my clients?		*The answers to these questions can only, really, be given by you, the reader, in relation to your service. These are my (the author's) reflections only.*
Can the results be applied to the local population of my practice and clients?	Yes	This study provides some useful evidence to support the development of a specific 'stroke' team within a Social Services department.

Contd

Table 3.2 *Contd.*

Question	Yes/no/ can't tell	Comments
Were all the important outcomes considered?	Can't tell/no	The lack of baseline functional measures is the major limitation of this evidence. The fact that the differences between the groups faded at the 6-month follow-up indicates that prompt intervention is interesting and should be explored further, especially in qualitative terms and the experience of post-stroke discharge from hospital should also be explored further.
Are the benefits of the intervention worth the harms and the costs?	Yes	A dedicated 'stroke' Social Services team would be costly to implement but would help to address the issue of waiting lists in many Social Services OT departments.

Are the results valid?

Did the trial address a clearly focused issue?

Was there a clearly stated aim to the research? Is the research attempting to address a clear research question? Does the research paper give a clear explanation of the population being studied? This question should include consideration of the criteria used for inclusion, and exclusion, of participants to the study. Does the paper give a clear overview of what interventions were being compared? Does the paper give a clear overview of the outcomes being measured and why those outcomes, and specific outcome measures, were chosen? At the end of reading the paper you should have a clear picture of who was being studied, what was being done to them and what the context of the study was.

Was the assignment of participants to treatments randomised?

The aim of this appraisal is to review RCTs. Therefore, a key question is whether participants were randomly assigned to the various groups. The paper should give a clear explanation of how the randomisation took place. If not, the paper is not a RCT and cannot be seen as 'gold standard' evidence.

Were all the participants who entered the trial properly accounted for at its conclusion?

Whilst *x* number of participants may begin the study it is usually the case that *y* number of participants complete the study, especially if there is a prolonged follow-up phase. Participants move on, change circumstances or die. However, it is important that all participants are accounted for in some way as part of the analysis. If the researchers fail to do this, the results may be biased.

The questions above should be used as a screening process to assess the overall value of the research. If the answers to these questions are negative the rigour of the research is questionable, and there will be little value in continuing to appraise the piece of research.

Is the literature review appropriate?

Does the literature provide a clear, comprehensive and up-to-date background to the research? Has literature been drawn from a wide range of sources? If the literature review is narrow and reliant on limited sources it may also reflect an underlying preconception and bias on the part of the researcher.

Were participants, health workers and study personnel 'blind' to the treatment?

Being 'blind' means being unaware of the nature of the research. One way of reducing potential bias or confounding influences is to ensure that the people involved in the research are blind. It would be unethical for participants to be unaware that they were part of a research programme. However, it is possible for participants to be unaware of whether they are in the intervention group or the control group. It is a well-accepted fact that if participants know they are part of a study this might influence their behaviour. This is known as the Hawthorne effect (DePoy & Gitlin, 1994; Bailey,

1997). The researchers, especially those carrying out any assessment or outcome measurement, should also be blind as the research process can influence them. The effect on the assessors is called the Rosenthal effect. However, the reader should also note that it may be difficult or unethical in some circumstances for those involved in the research to be blind to the nature of the research.

Were the groups similar at the start of the trial?

The premise of randomisation is that all variables are equally distributed between the groups. The groups should, therefore, be similar in terms of relevant factors such as age, gender, social class, ethnicity, length of stay in hospital, etc., as well as for the study's baseline measures. Statistical analysis should be used to establish that there are no significant differences between the groups, and detailed demographic and baseline profiles of the groups should be presented as part of the results.

Apart from the experimental intervention, were the groups treated equally?

This question relates to two aspects of the research. Firstly, how many people were involved in giving the intervention to the intervention group? If more than one person was involved, was the process of intervention clearly standardised between the different personnel? The second aspect relates to how the control group was treated. If the control group was receiving the 'usual' or 'normal' intervention, was this standardised? Differences in intervention within the various study groups may act as a confounding factor to influence the results.

Were ethical issues considered?

Ethical issues include informed consent, confidentiality, risk factors, denial or withholding treatment, or distress caused to the participants. The researchers should discuss how these issues have been dealt with within the study.

What are the results?

Was there an adequate description of the data collection methods used?

The process of data collection should be clearly described. Were the measures used in the study valid and reliable tools for assessing the relevant outcomes? All outcome measures should be referenced and a review of their validity and reliability should be given. If new measures have been developed and used in the study, have these been subjected to a rigorous assessment of their reliability and validity?

Were the methods of analysis appropriate, clearly described and justified?

Did the analysis relate to the aims and research questions? Was the choice of statistical analysis explained with a clear rationale for the choice of tests?

What are the key findings?

Do these results answer the research questions? Each outcome measure should be analysed and the results presented, with clear comparisons between the groups.

How significant were the results?

If there are significant differences between the groups, how large are the differences? If confidence intervals are given, how narrow are they?

How will the results help me work with my clients?

Can the results be applied to the local population of my practice and clients?

Consider the nature of the study's participants, how similar are they to your client group? If the study is of in-patients, how well can this be applied to an out-patient or community setting? Do you have the skills necessary to use the intervention or do you need further skills and training?

Were all the important outcomes considered?

Any research can only measure a limited number of outcomes. However, has the research measured the outcomes you feel are the most relevant? If other outcomes should have been considered, do you need to find more evidence before changing your current intervention?

Are the benefits of the intervention worth the harms and the costs?

The paper may not address this question. However, you will need to consider the implications of changing your practice, not only for yourself but also for your clients and your purchasers.

Activity

- Identify a RCT relevant to your area of practice/interest
- Using the appraisal questions above, work with a colleague to appraise the article and to assess its value as evidence

Further reading

The following references will allow the reader to explore the nature and scope of experimental research in more depth.

Bailey, D.M. (1997) *Research for the Health Professional*, 2nd edn. Philadelphia: FA Davis Co.

DePoy, E. & Gitlin, L.N. (1994) *Introduction to Research*. St Louis: Mosby.

Greenhalgh, T. (1997) *How to Read a Paper*. London: BMJ Publishing Group.

Munro, B.H. & Page, E.B. (1993) *Statistical Methods for Health Care Research*. Philadelphia: J.B. Lippincott Co.

Pereira-Maxwell, F (1998). *A–Z of Medical Statistics: A Comparison for Critical Appraisal.* London: Arnold.

Robson, C. (1993) *Real World Research*. Oxford: Blackwell Publishers.

Chapter 4
SYSTEMATIC REVIEWS

Whilst randomised controlled trials (RCTs) are the 'gold standard' for evidence, as we have seen in Chapter 3, the results of a RCT may not be significant or may be statistically significant without being *clinically* significant. The problem with many RCTs is that they are based on small numbers of participants and the likelihood, therefore, of a highly significant result is reduced. However, if the findings from a number of RCTs can be combined and re-analysed, the results may be far more clinically significant and the evidence of the effectiveness of the intervention becomes much stronger. This is the purpose and value of systematic reviews and meta-analyses. In the hierarchy of evidence (see Chapter 1), systematic reviews and meta-analysis of RCTs are at the top of the hierarchy and form the highest level of evidence.

Systematic reviews and meta-analyses of OT interventions are relatively rare, at the moment. A search of AMED using the search:

'systematic review AND occupational therapy'

produced no hits. A similar search using:

'meta-analysis AND occupational therapy'

produced only two hits (Cusick, 1986; Carlson *et al*., 1996). AMED was then re-searched using:

'systematic review'

and

'systematic AND review'.

The 'systematic review' search produced 16 hits, whilst the 'systematic AND review' search produced 37 hits. All of the first 16 hits were repeated in the second, 'systematic AND review' search. Of these 37 hits, only five were of any relevance to the evidence-based OT and three of these references dealt with methodological issues within systematic reviews. Only Langhorne *et al*. (1996) and Droogan and Bannigan (1997) are actual reviews of evidence which might be of interest to the evidence-based OT. A broad search, using 'meta-analysis' resulted in 69 hits, of which some 19 (including Cusick, 1986; Carlson *et al*. 1996) had potential value for the evidence-based OT.

A search of the Cochrane Library was more successful. A search using the medical subject heading (MeSH) term 'occupational therapy' revealed two hits on the DARE: Abstracts of Quality Assessed Systematic Reviews listing. This gave reviews of the Carlson *et al*. (1996) meta-analysis of the effectiveness of OT with older people and a review of the use of occupationally embedded exercise by Lin *et al*. (1997). The DARE reviews give a succinct overview and appraisal of the aims, process and findings of any review, as well as an evaluation of the quality of the review. A 'simple' search of the Cochrane Library using 'occupational therapy' produced nine hits on DARE and 34 hits on the Cochrane Database of Systematic Review. The Cochrane Database hits included 21 completed reviews and 13 protocols. Not all of the reviews were of relevance, however reviews of note included:

Community mental health teams (CMHT) for severe mental illness
Falls prevention in the elderly
Hip fracture: in-patient rehabilitation
Hospital at home
Life skills programmes and schizophrenia
(Reality orientation) RO in dementia
Reminiscence therapy (RT) in dementia.

Protocols of interest, for reviews currently being conducted, included:

Cognitive behaviour therapy in schizophrenia
Cognitive rehabilitation in schizophrenia
Counselling in primary care
Day hospital treatment for psychiatric disorders
Guidelines for professions allied to medicine (PAMS)
Rheumatoid arthritis (RA): dynamic exercise therapy

As well as demonstrating the somewhat limited number of systematic reviews available to the evidence-based OT, these searches have also added to the lessons learnt in Chapter 2. The AMED search demonstrated the value of using Boolean operators, such as AND, to expand search terms, whilst the Cochrane search demonstrated the limitations of relying solely on MeSH terms at the expense of natural language.

Whilst systematic reviews and meta-analyses are relatively rare in OT at the moment, in spite of Ottenbacher's (1983) support, they are sources of the highest level of evidence. This chapter will discuss the nature of systematic reviews and meta-analyses. The ways of presenting data and findings in systematic reviews and meta-analyses will be outlined, with relevant examples (given as Boxes) as illustrations. The chapter will conclude by outlining how systematic reviews can be appraised and used to answer evidence-based questions.

Overview of systematic reviews

All researchers know the value of reviewing the existing literature on a given topic. These surveys of existing literature often lead to narrative or qualitative reviews of the literature. This is where the research findings for a given topic are presented in some form of overview format. The various studies and their findings are often presented in table format. However, little attempt is made to re-analyse the findings within a qualitative review. This may be because a variety of research techniques have been employed and direct comparisons cannot be made. A further limitation of the narrative review is that there is often subjectivity involved in the selection of the articles for inclusion or exclusion from the review (Cusick,

1986). Whilst narrative reviews can provide interesting food for thought, they rarely provide high-quality evidence.

Systematic reviews aim to improve upon narrative and qualitative reviews by using rigorous methods to find and review research evidence. Langhorne and Dennis (1998) proposed three roles for systematic reviews:

- To provide the most reliable summary of available information and research on a given intervention
- To provide invaluable pointers for future research
- Reviews may also provide the best estimate of whether a particular intervention is effective

The aim of any systematic review is to synthesise the findings of all the available, appropriate, evidence and to do so scientifically, rigorously and without bias. As with all research, systematic reviews follow a clear process (Mulrow & Oxman, 1997; de Vet *et al.* 1997; Langhorne & Dennis, 1998).

The systematic review should begin with a clear objective and research question; this will guide and frame the review. If the question is too broad the reviewers may be overwhelmed with research that is difficult to synthesise and interpret. If the topic is too narrow this may result in limited numbers of RCTs being identified and an inability to draw clear conclusions.

Box 4.1

Three systematic reviews will be used as illustrations throughout this chapter. One review (Carlson *et al.*, 1996) is an OT review. The other two reviews are Cochrane Reviews (Spector & Orrell, 1998a,b).

Both Carlson *et al.* (1996) and Spector and Orrell (1998a) are broad reviews. Carlson *et al.* (1996) were looking at the effectiveness of OT in treating older people, whilst Spector and Orrell (1998a) were looking at the effectiveness of reminiscence therapy (RT) with older people with dementia.

Spector and Orrell's (1998b) review of reality orientation (RO) was more focused, as it looked specifically at classroom-based RO with older people with dementia.

Having defined the question, the reviewers must then carry out a comprehensive search of all potentially relevant sources of information. This should ensure that all relevant RCTs are located and can be included in the review. Searches should include both computer and hand searches. Relevant databases and Internet sites should be identified for computer searches. A comprehensive search strategy, including the identification of key terms, should be developed for the computer searches. Relevant journals, conference proceedings and current awareness literature should be identified for hand searching. Other relevant sources of information, such as specialist libraries and specialists and experts in the relevant fields, should also be identified.

Box 4:2

Carlson *et al.* (1996) hand searched a range of OT journals and computer searched MEDLINE, using the search terms:

OT and
Geriatric
Gerontic
Gerontology
Gerentological
Elderly
Elders
Older
Aged

and identified 53 potential references.

Spector and Orrell (1998a,b) identified similar sources for both their searches. They used the terms:

Reality orientation
Dementia
Controlled study
Trial

for their RO review (1998a), and the terms:

Reminiscence therapy
Dementia
Control*
Trial or study

for their RT search (1998b). Their computer searched a range of sources, including:

MEDLINE
PsychLit
OMNI
BIDS
Dissertation Abstracts International

Journals (e.g. *Aging and Mental Health, Journal of Gerontology*), conference proceedings (e.g. British Psychological Society), Web sites and the Alzheimer's Disease Society library were hand searched. Specialists in the field were also contacted. Forty-three publications were identified in the RO search and 15 publications in the RT search.

A review protocol should be developed. This will outline the criteria to be used for deciding whether studies will be included or excluded from the review. The criteria should include the types of participants, the types of interventions, the outcome measures, the types of studies and the methodological quality criteria. The protocol should ensure that bias is reduced by explicitly outlining the inclusion and exclusion criteria. The use of methodological quality criteria also ensures the rigour of the review and the inclusion of high-quality RCT evidence.

Box 4.3

The inclusion criteria used by Carlson *et al.* (1996) were:

- Publication between 1979 and 1994
- OT intervention to 4+ subjects with a mean age of 60+
- Inclusion of statistical information, e.g. means, SD
- Outcomes relevant to policymakers, e.g. health, function, well-being

The criteria for both the Spector and Orrell (1998a,b) reviews were more detailed. For the RO review (1998b) the criteria included:

- *Participants* – age 55+, diagnosis of dementia
- *Intervention* – at least 10 sessions over a minimum 3-week period, 4+ participants for each group
- *Outcomes* – cognitive and behaviour measures, well-recognised published tests
- *Studies* – RCTs

Using the inclusion/exclusion criteria, trials should then be selected or rejected. In order to reduce bias, this process should be carried out by more than one reviewer. All excluded trials should be listed within the review, with the reasons for exclusion outlined. Of the initial 52 publications identified by Carlson *et al*. (1996) only 14 met their inclusion criteria, whilst in the RO review (Spector & Orrell, 1998b) of the initial 43 publications only eight met the inclusion criteria and for the RT review (Spector & Orrell, 1998a), of the initial 15 publications only three met the inclusion criteria. The methodological quality of the included trials is then appraised.

Having identified and appraised the relevant and appropriate trials, the next stage is to extract and synthesise the data. Various methods of data synthesis are available to the systematic reviewer. However, it is not the task of this chapter to review these methods. The outcomes of data synthesis will be discussed in the next section of this chapter (Understanding the numbers in systematic reviews). The final stage of the systematic review process is to interpret the findings, drawing in all the available evidence.

Whilst systematic reviews aim to provide the least biased and most reliable summary of available evidence, they are not without their limitations. The main areas of limitation and bias in systematic reviews are: publication bias, study quality, and the diversity of studies. Publication bias, and the tendency to publish only interesting and positive results, has already been mentioned in the discussion of RCTs in Chapter 3. Systematic reviews endeavour to overcome publication bias by accessing information from unpublished sources, theses and conferences where neutral or non-significant findings may be discussed.

Systematic reviews are only as good as the primary data they re-analyse. Not all systematic reviews are rigorous about the methodological quality criteria used to include and exclude studies. A famous criticism of systematic reviews was proposed by Eysenck (1978: 517):

> 'a mass of reports – good, bad, and indifferent – are fed into the computer . . . "garbage in – garbage out".'

Interestingly, both Cusick (1986) and de Vet *et al*. (1997) argue that the inclusion of poor quality studies may not affect the outcome of a meta-analysis.

Diversity is the final area of limitation and potential bias in systematic reviews. The nature of systematic reviews is that the results of a number of studies are compared. However, the similarities and diversity of the various studies must be considered in terms of the following questions:

- How similar are the participants in each study?
- What is the context of the various trials?
  - Can studies from different countries be compared?
  - Can studies of in-patient and out-patient settings and interventions be compared?
- How comparable are the various interventions?

It might be possible to justify the homogeneity (similarity) of the various study populations or, if there is evidence of heterogeneity (differences), it might be necessary to compare sub-groups within the populations or to take the heterogeneity into account in the data analysis.

Understanding the numbers in systematic reviews

The main task of any meta-analysis is to take each trial and compare the number of participants in the intervention group who had a successful outcome with the number of participants in the control group who had a successful outcome. Each comparison can then be totalled together to give an overall *effects* score. However, the analysis is not quite as simple as this makes it sound. It is often impossible to calculate a simple comparison because the numbers of participants in the intervention group and the control group vary. The comparison is, therefore, usually expressed in terms of an *odds ratio* (OR) (Langhorne & Dennis, 1998; Pereira-Maxwell, 1998). As Box 4.4 illustrates, other measures are also used in meta-analysis.

An OR is a number that expresses the ratio of the likelihood (odds) of a particular outcome (e.g. improved function, death, level of independence) occurring amongst the participants in the intervention group in comparison with the likelihood (odds) of that outcome occurring in the control group. It should be noted that, somewhat perversely, ORs are usually expressed in terms of the prevention of a bad outcome (e.g. death, dependence) rather than in terms of a positive outcome (e.g. improved function). An OR of 1 indicates that there is the same likelihood (odds) of the outcome occurring in both the intervention group and the control group. An OR of *less than* 1 indicates a better outcome in the intervention group, or evidence for the effectiveness of the intervention. An OR of *more than* 1 indicates better outcomes in the control group, or no evidence for the effectiveness of the intervention. Odds ratios are always shown with a confidence interval (CI), usually of 95% (see Chapter 3 for a discussion of confidence intervals). Confidence intervals are included because the OR is not an accurate estimate of the 'true' value for the population and so 95%CI gives the best estimation of the possible range of odds.

The results of a meta-analysis are usually presented in a table format where the results of each trial are presented and the overall total is given at the bottom of the table. Figure 4.1 is an example of meta-analysis results from Langhorne and Dennis' (1998) review of the effectiveness of stroke units. Because of the number of black squares or dots (blobs) in the table, these tables are often referred to as *blobbograms*. The blob (or black square) represents the odds ratio for the particular trial and the horizontal line represents the 95%CI for that OR. This line is often referred to as the *wobble factor* as it represents the uncertainty and possible variation of the OR. The vertical line down the table is known as *the line of no effect* and represents an OR of 1. Thus, trials with a blob to the right of the vertical line (e.g. Tampere in Fig. 4.1) indicate a more favourable outcome in the control group. Trials where the potential (wobble) outcome, as indicated by the 95%CI, *might* be in favour of the control group (e.g. Birmingham in Fig. 4.1) are shown with a confidence interval line that crosses the line of no effect.

In Fig. 4.1 the information given in the table includes:

- The name of the study
- The number of participants in the intervention group (Expt) with an adverse result (n) in comparison to the total number of participants in the intervention group (N)
- Similar data for the control group (Ctrl)
- Graphic representation of the odds ratio (OR) and 95% confidence interval (95%CI)
- The actual numerical data for the odds ratio and 95%CI

Comparison: Organised stroke unit care vs conventional care
Outcome: Death or dependency by the end of scheduled follow-up

Study	Expt n/N	Ctrl n/N	OR (95%CI Fixed)	OR (95%CI Fixed)
Birmingham	8/29	9/23		0.59 [0.18, 1.91]
Dover	65/116	79/117		0.61 [0.36, 1.04]
Edinburgh	93/155	94/156		0.99 [0.63, 1.56]
Helsinki	47/121	65/122		0.56 [0.33, 0.93]
Illinois	20/56	17/35		0.59 [0.25, 1.39]
Kuopio	31/50	31/45		0.74 [0.31, 1.73]
Montreal	58/65	60/65		0.69 [0.21, 2.30]
New York	23/42	23/40		0.89 [0.37, 2.14]
Newcastle	26/34	28/33		0.58 [0.17, 2.00]
Nottingham	123/176	100/139		0.91 [0.55, 1.48]
Orpington (1993)	101/124	108/121		0.53 [0.25, 1.10]
Orpington (1995)	34/34	37/37		0.92 [0.02, 47.65]
Perth	10/29	14/30		0.60 [0.21, 1.72]
Tampere	53/98	55/113		1.24 [0.72, 2.14]
Trondheim	54/110	81/110		0.35 [0.20, 0.61]
Umeå	52/110	102/183		0.71 [0.44, 1.14]
Uppsala	45/60	41/52		0.80 [0.33, 1.95]
Total (95%CI)	**843/1409**	**944/1421**		**0.71 [0.60, 0.84]**

Fig. 4.1 Example of meta-analysis results. For an explanation of abbreviations used see text. Meta-analysis comparing stroke unit care with conventional care: death or dependency at the end of follow-up (median 1 year: range 6 weeks to 1 year). (Reproduced with permission from Langhorne, P. & Dennis, M. (1998) *Stroke Units: An Evidence Based Approach*, p.44. London: BMJ Publishing Group.

At the bottom of the table is the total result for the review represented with a diamond. The centre of the diamond is the total OR and the width of the diamond shows the 95% CI for the total OR.

According to Fig. 4.1, the Montreal study had 65 participants in both the intervention and the control groups. Of the 65 patients treated on a stroke unit (the experimental group) 58 were either dead or dependent (as opposed to independent, measured on an activities of daily living [ADL] score) by the end of the follow-up period. Of the 65 patients who were treated on a conventional care ward, 60 were dead or dependent by the end of the follow-up. When converted to an OR this gives a result of 0.69, which is in favour of the intervention, and a 95%CI of OR from 0.21 to 2.30, indicating a degree of wobble from favouring stroke unit care to favouring conventional care. The total results, however, indicate in favour of stroke units with a total OR of 0.71 and a 95%CI from 0.60 to 0.84; all of these values are on the intervention side of the line of no effect. From these findings it might be safe to conclude that stroke units are effective not only in preventing death but also in reducing the level of dependence

Box 4.4

Spector and Orrell's (1998a) review of RO presented their results under two headings, cognition and behaviour, and presented the results in terms of the *mean difference* between the groups. For mean differences, 0 = no difference and a negative score favours the intervention. In terms of cognition, the mean difference was –0.586 with a 95%CI of –0.952 to –0.220. For behaviour the mean difference was –0.659 with a 95%CI of –1.268 to –0.050. Both of these results indicate evidence for the effectiveness of RO.

Spector and Orrell's (1998b) review of RT also used mean differences for cognition and behaviour. For cognition the mean difference was 0.049 with a 95%CI of –4.371 to 4.771. This result favours the control group. For behaviour the results were a mean difference of –3.3 with a 95%CI of –14.190 to 7.590, which slightly favours the intervention. From this review there appears to be little support for the effectiveness of RT from the limited number of studies analysed.

Carlson *et al.*'s (1996) review of OT with older people used *mean effect size* and a 90%CI to present their results. As with ORs a value of less than 1 indicates a result favouring the intervention. The overall mean effect size for all the interventions reviewed was 0.51 with a 90% CI of 0.27–0.75. Interventions were then reviewed separately with the following results:

- ADL – mean effect size: 0.67, 90%CI from 0.08 to 1.26
- Physical health – mean effect size: 0.32, 90%CI from 0.09 to 0.55
- Psychosocial well-being – mean effect size: 0.37, 90%CI from 0.20 to 0.54

These results indicate overall evidence for the effectiveness of OT with older people. However, when the interventions are reviewed separately, whilst the evidence is mostly in favour of the effectiveness of OT, the evidence for the effectiveness of OT for improving ADL function is somewhat equivocal.

Appraising systematic reviews

As with any appraisal, the appraisal of a systematic review addresses three main questions:

- Are the results valid?
- What are the results?
- How will these results help me work with my clients?

Table 4.1 gives an overview of the questions to ask when appraising a systematic review. These questions are based on the questions developed as part of the Critical Appraisal Skills Programme (CASP) initiative with some additions which the author felt were relevant to evidence-based OT (see Chapter 7 for more information about the CASP initiative).

The reader will note that there are similarities in the questions asked to appraise any piece of research, be it a RCT, a qualitative study or a systematic review. The various questions will now be expanded within the context of appraising a systematic review. Table 4.2 contains a worked example of a critical appraisal of a systematic review (Carlson *et al.* 1996).

Table 4.1 Questions to ask when critically appraising a systematic review.

Are the results valid?

- Did the review address a clearly focused issue?
- Do you think the important, relevant studies were included?
- Did the reviewers establish clear inclusion and exclusion criteria for the identified studies?
- Did the review's authors do enough to assess the methodological quality of the included studies?
- If the results of the review have been combined, was it reasonable to do so?

What are the results?

- Were the methods of meta-analysis appropriate and clearly justified?
- What is the overall result of the review?
- How precise are the results?

How will these results help me work with my clients?

- Can the results be applied to the local population of my practice and clients?
- Were all important outcomes considered?
- Are the benefits worth the harms and the costs?

Are the results valid?

Did the review address a clearly focused issue?

As with the appraisal of RCTs or qualitative research, the first question to ask when appraising a systematic review is whether the review has a clear aim and research question. If the aim is broad, have the reviewers asked smaller, subsidiary questions? Did the reviewers clearly establish the parameters of the review question in terms of the population to be included, the interventions to be reviewed and compared, and the outcomes being measured?

This question can be used as a screening process to help you to decide whether it is worth spending precious reading time on a particular review. If the answers to this question are negative it is probably not worth continuing to read and appraise the review, as it will provide poor-quality evidence of effectiveness.

Table 4.2 Worked example of a critical appraisal of a systematic review using: Carlson, M., Fanchiang, S.P., Zemke, R. & Clark, F. (1996) A meta-analysis of the effectiveness of occupational therapy for older persons. *American Journal of Occupational Therapy*, **50**(2), 89–98.

Question	Yes/no/ can't tell	Comments
Are the results valid?		
Did the review address a clearly focused issue?	Yes/no	The answer to this question could be open to some debate. The review does have a clear focus: To examine the degree of effectiveness of OT interventions with older people. Effectiveness was seen in terms of enhancing the psychosocial well-being, function, and physical health of older people. However, this is a very broad topic and the review could be seen as covering too wide an area to be useful as evidence.
If the answer to this screening question is 'yes', is it worth carrying on with the appraisal?	Yes	Although the answer to the screening question was equivocal, there is so little evidence of the effectiveness of OT interventions that you have decided to proceed with the appraisal.
Do you think the important, relevant studies were included?	Yes	The published literature was extensively searched with hand searching of a range of OT journals and computer searching of MEDLINE using a range of key words. The references included in all potentially useful articles were also scanned for additional studies. However, no attempt was made to search the grey literature which could mean that potentially useful studies were not accessed.
Did the reviewers establish clear inclusion and exclusion criteria for the identified studies?	Yes	Four inclusion criteria were utilised and justified: • Publication between 1979 and 1994

Contd

Table 4.2 *Contd.*

Question	Yes/no/ can't tell	Comments
		• The study must be of an OT intervention, with 4+ subjects, with a mean age of 60+ • The study must include a quantitative evaluation of effectiveness • The outcomes should be of relevance to policymakers The reasons why certain studies were rejected, based on the inclusion/exclusion criteria, are clearly outlined. However, it is not clear whether more than one of the authors was involved in the inclusion/exclusion screening and so inclusion/exclusion bias cannot be completely ruled out.
Did the review's authors do enough to assess the methodological quality of the included studies?	No	There appears to be no evidence of any assessment of the methodological quality of the studies included in the review. Thus the review should be viewed with some caution as the meta-analysis may be affected by the inclusion of research which is of poor methodological quality.
If the results of the review have been combined, was it reasonable to do so?	Yes/no	The answer to this question is open to considerable debate. The range of interventions and outcome measures used in this review are very varied and diverse, although they all relate to OT. Whilst all OT outcomes might be related in general terms, is it methodologically sound to compare outcomes as diverse as ADL scores, life satisfaction ratings and finger dexterity?

Contd

Table 4.2 *Contd.*

Question	Yes/no/ can't tell	Comments
What are the results?		
Were the methods of meta-analysis appropriate and clearly justified?	Yes	Effect size estimates were calculated by two independent assessors. The process of data extraction and analysis was explained and clearly justified.
What is the overall result of the review?	—	The individual characteristics and effect size for each of the included studies is clearly presented in table format. The overall results (with statistical analysis) are presented in terms of: • All included studies • RCTs only • ADL outcomes • Physical health outcomes • Psychosocial well-being outcomes. Measures of clinical significance are not included in the data analysis.
How precise are the results?	—	The results show significant difference for all interventions. The levels of significance vary from $P < 0.05$ for physical health outcomes to $P < 0.001$ for all other results. Confidence intervals (at the 90% level) are given for all results. However, the CI for ADL function is rather wide and crosses the line of no effect (0.08–1.26). Thus, although there is evidence for the effectiveness of all OT interventions with older people, the evidence for ADL function is rather weak.

Contd

Table 4.2 *Contd.*

Question	Yes/no/ can't tell	Comments
How will these results help me work with my clients?		*The answers to these questions can only, really, be given by you, the reader, in relation to your service. These are my (the author's) reflections only.*
Can the results be applied to the local population of my practice and clients?	yes/no	Because of the breadth of interventions included in this review, it could be argued that this paper provides useful evidence for any OT services working with older clients. However, the very breadth of the study is its chief limitation. By addressing the whole of OT with older people it has become too diverse and provides little useful evidence.
Were all important outcomes considered?	Can't tell/no	The diversity of the review has been mentioned above. The other area of concern is the lack of quality assessment of the included papers. Thus any evidence of the effectiveness of OT with older people provided by this paper must be flawed by the inclusion of potentially flawed data.
Are the benefits worth the harms and the costs?	No	The breadth of the paper does not allow this question to be adequately addressed.

Do you think the important, relevant studies were included?

As we have seen, studies need to be gathered from a range of sources. Have the reviewers given full details of the search strategy, including the key words used? Were these adequate and appropriate to the topic? Have the reviewers searched a range of databases? Knowing that not all research is published, have the reviewers made efforts to find unpublished research? Have the reviewers followed up reference lists and contacted experts and specialists in the appropriate fields?

Did the reviewers establish clear inclusion and exclusion criteria for identified studies?

Having identified relevant studies, how did the reviewers approach the task of deciding which studies to include or exclude from the review? Did the reviewers outline the criteria they used? To avoid bias, was more than one person involved in inclusion/exclusion decisions? Have details of excluded studies and the reasons for exclusion been given?

Did the review's authors do enough to assess the methodological quality of the included studies?

As well as giving criteria for inclusion and exclusion, the reviewers should also outline the criteria used for appraising the quality of the research to be included in the review. There is little value in reviewing poor quality or flawed research evidence. The task of appraising the methodological quality should, like inclusion and exclusion, be a shared task with more than one reviewer, independently, appraising the methodological rigour of the various papers.

If the results of the review have been combined, was it reasonable to do so?

The characteristics of the various included studies should be presented, probably in table format, to allow you to judge whether the studies are similar enough to allow comparisons to be made. Were the study designs similar? Were the interventions similar? Have similar outcome measures been used? If there is evidence of heterogeneity, has this been accounted for in the statistical analysis?

What are the results?

Were the methods of meta-analysis appropriate and clearly justified?

Various methods are used for meta-analysis. Has the process of data extraction and analysis been clearly explained and justified? Do the methods used appear to be appropriate for the various studies and types of data?

What is the overall result of the review?

Does the overall result of the review address the research question? If the review asked subsidiary questions, have these been answered by the results? Have overall results been given for the various outcome measures? Has the statistical significance of any differences between interventions been tested? Have measures of clinical significance been used?

How precise are the results?

Have results been presented with confidence intervals? Is the confidence interval used (e.g. 90%, 95%) appropriate?

How will these results help me work with my clients?

Can the results be applied to the local population of my practice and clients?

Consider the nature of the population covered by the reviewed trials, how similar is it to your client group? Can the findings be applied to your particular setting? Are the review population and your client group similar enough?

Were all important outcomes considered?

A review is only as broad as its original parameters, some outcomes will not be assessed. However, does the review cover all the outcomes you are concerned with?

Are the benefits worth the harms and the costs?

The review may include some form of cost/benefit discussion, but if not, what do you think? Is the strength of the intervention worth any possible costs or harms?

Gray (1997) argued that systematic reviews are the best source of evidence for health care decision and policy makers. However, he does add the note of caution that the quality of systematic reviews is variable. Any systematic review should be appraised carefully before any judgements are made.

Activity

- Identify a systematic review of relevance to your area of practice/ interest
- Using the appraisal questions above, work with a colleague to appraise the article and to assess its value as evidence
- The Cochrane Library is a major source of information on systematic reviews; spend some time exploring the Cochrane Library Database of Systematic Reviews

Further reading

The following readings will allow the reader to explore the value and use of systematic reviews and meta-analysis in more depth.

Chalmers, I. & Altman, D.G. (eds) (1995). *Systematic Reviews*. London: BMJ Publishing Group.

Cusick, A. (1986) Research in occupational therapy: meta-analysis. *Australian Occupational Therapy Journal* **33**(4), 142–7.

Greenhalgh, T. (1997) *How to Read a Paper*. London: BMJ Publishing Group.

Hayes, R.L. (1998) Evidence-based practice: the Cochrane Collaboration, and occupational therapy. *Canadian Journal of Occupational Therapy*, **65**(3), 144–51.

Langhorne, P. & Dennis, M. (1998) *Stroke Units: An Evidence Based Approach*. London: BMJ Publishing Group.

McKinnell, I. & Elliott, J. (1997) *The Cochrane Library: Self-Training Guide and Notes*. Oxford: Anglia and Oxford NHS Executive Anglia & Oxford. http://www.lib.jr2.ox.ac.uk/nhserdd/aordd/evidence/clibtrng.htm

Mulrow, C.D. (1994) Rationale for systematic reviews. *British Medical Journal* **309**, 597–9.

Mulrow, C.D. & Oxman, A.D. (eds) (1997) *Cochrane Collaboration Handbook* [updated September, 1997]. In: The Cochrane Library [database on disk and CD-ROM]. The Cochrane Collaboration. Oxford: Update Software; 1994, issue 4.

Sinclair, A. & Dickinson, E. (1998) *Effective Practice in Rehabilitation*. London: King's Fund.

Chapter 5
QUALITATIVE RESEARCH AS EVIDENCE

Qualitative research has, for some time, been seen as the methodology of choice for OT research (Kielhofner, 1982; Krefting, 1989a; Yerxa, 1991). However it is interesting to note that a search of AMED using

'qualitative research AND occupational therapy'

produced only 12 hits, whilst searches using specific qualitative research approaches as the search terms produced further, relevant hits. The terms:

'phenomenol* AND occupational therapy'

(phenomenol* was truncated to access both 'phenomenology' and 'phenomenological') produced 11 hits, and:

'ethnography'

produced a further nine possible articles. The lack of success of the AMED search probably reflects more on the indexing in AMED than on the use of qualitative research in OT.

Qualitative research has, until recently, had a less prominent place in evidence-based practice. Qualitative research is often, wrongly, viewed as lacking validity and reliability. Numbers, and anything that can be quantified, are acceptable as 'scientific' fact and, therefore, as evidence. Ideas and words are seen as biased and unscientific and, therefore, of limited value as evidence. As Greenhalgh (1997) pointed out, even 'facts' which have little evidence to support them are accepted, because of the apparent evidence of the numbers.

Qualitative research is beginning to be seen as acceptable and appropriate as evidence to answer certain questions. Qualitative research is even becoming 'trendy' (Greenhalgh, 1997) in health care research. More and more health care researchers are realising that randomised controlled trials (RCTs) do not answer all the relevant questions. Qualitative research generates deeper, richer data, which can address issues of quality and the client's experience of health care. In the previous chapter on systematic reviews, we saw how stroke units can be effective in reducing disability. What this research cannot tell us is why stroke units are more effective than other, equally rehabilitation-orientated, medical units.

A Cochrane Collaboration working group is currently working to develop criteria for appraising qualitative research and using qualitative research within systematic reviews (Popay *et al.*, 1997; Popay & Williams, 1998). Qualitative research has played a major role in OT for some time and is beginning to be seen as an important and valuable source of evidence within health care. Evidence-based OTs should find qualitative research a rich source of valuable evidence and should provide reflexivity on their interventions and practice.

This chapter will give a brief overview of research from a qualitative perspective, beginning by outlining the methodology, approaches and methods of qualitative research. As in earlier chapters, relevant examples (presented as Boxes) will be given to illustrate these points. The chapter will then explore the often contentious issue of how qualitative research can be seen as 'good' research. The chapter will then conclude with an overview of how the evidence-based OT can appraise qualitative research as evidence for the effectiveness of interventions and practice. As with the previous two chapters, examples of 'real' OT research will be used to illustrate various points.

Overview of qualitative research

Research is often seen as being divided into two *methodologies* or philosophical paradigms. These differing, and for some opposing, methodologies are qualitative and quantitative research. Having identified the research methodology, all research can then be divided into particular research *approaches*. Research approaches in quantitative research include:

- Experiments
- RCTs
- Surveys

Research approaches in qualitative research include:

- Phenomenology
- Ethnography
- Grounded theory

Within any research approach a variety of research *methods* can be used to gather the actual data for the study. These research methods include:

- Measurement
- Observation
- Interviews
- Diaries

Qualitative methodology

Qualitative and quantitative research are often seen as being diametrically opposed (DePoy & Gitlin, 1994). Whilst qualitative and quantitative research are based on radically different philosophical paradigms, both methodologies are ways of viewing the process of empirical investigation. Table 5.1 summarises the differences between the two methodologies (Krefting, 1989a; DePoy & Gitlin, 1994; Bailey, 1997; Greenhalgh, 1997).

Table 5.1 Overview of the differences between qualitative and quantitative methodology.

Parameter	*Qualitative methodology*	*Quantitative methodology*
Philosophical background	Realism/existentialism	Rationalism/positivism
Philosophical approach	Holistic	Reductionist
Academic fields	Sociology, anthropology, social psychology	Natural sciences, medicine, psychology
Reasoning	Inductive	Deductive
Mode of enquiry	Naturalistic enquiry	Scientific method
Perspective	Emic (insider) Subjective	Etic (outsider) Objective
Research question	Explores a research question Describes and understands a setting or phenomenon	Test a hypothesis Demonstrates cause and effect
Research process	Researcher is inside the research setting Definitions evolve with the research Flexible approach	Researcher stands outside the research setting Specific operational definitions are established Control Clearly defined process
Data	Words Subjective Observations Interviews Content analysis	Numbers Measurement Objective Statistical analysis
Rigour	Trustworthiness	Validity and reliability

The aim of quantitative research in health care (RCTs, systematic reviews) is to provide statistical evidence to evaluate the effectiveness of particular interventions whereas the aim of qualitative research is to explore phenomena in their natural settings, to explore the meanings and interpretations people bring to their everyday lives and experiences, and to explore the complexities of human life and behaviour (Denzin & Lincoln, 1994). Quantitative research can often strip the context and the humanity away from the focus and setting of the research. For qualitative research, context is vitally important. In health and social care terms, qualitative research can address such questions as:

- What stops people giving up smoking? (Greenhalgh, 1997)
- What is it like to live with the aftermath of traumatic head injury? (Krefting, 1989b)
- What makes any activity meaningful? (Taylor & McGruder, 1996)

Box 5:1

Munroe (1996) used a qualitative methodology to study the nature and scope of clinical reasoning in community OT. She observed and interviewed 30 community OTs. Data were gathered about the content and meaning of the therapists' thinking during their routine interactions with clients. The data were coded and categorised and it was found that the therapists used a variety of reasoning patterns.

Qualitative research approaches

Qualitative research can be used to 'understand the meanings, experiences, and phenomena as they evolve in the natural setting, (DePoy & Gitlin, 1994: 48). This can be done from a variety of different perspectives, by asking different types of research questions. The different perspectives and research questions will need to be explored using different research approaches.

Ethnography aims to describe a culture (Krefting, 1989a; DePoy & Gitlin, 1994; Bailey, 1997). Ethnography has been used within anthropology to describe and interpret cultural patterns of groups, to understand cultural meanings and to understand how people organise and interpret their experience. The sorts of research questions asked in ethnographic studies are, broadly, 'what is happening here and why is it happening?'

Box 5.2

Examples of OT ethnographic studies include:

Townsend's (1996) study of mental health OT practice. She posed the question 'what are the possibilities and constraints for OTs to enable the empowerment of adults who attend mental health day programs?' She explored this issue using an institutional ethnographic process.

Spencer *et al.'s* (1995) study of the life of a patient following spinal cord injury and how he learnt the culture of rehabilitation and being a disabled person.

Bailey (1997) proposed that successful ethnography helps the reader to behave appropriately in the particular cultural setting, whether the setting is a mental health care facility, rehabilitation unit, or day care centre for clients with dementia (Hasselkus, 1992).

Phenomenological research aims to explore the lived experience of individuals. Particular phenomena (or events, or experiences) are explored in an attempt to understand how individuals interpret and give meaning to their lives. Whereas ethnography can involve interpretation and critical analysis on the part of the researcher, meaning and interpretation within phenomenology is drawn from the participants. Phenomenological research, therefore, unlike ethnography, cannot be generalised. The insights and understandings of individuals' experience gained from phenomenological research can, however, be used as tools to reflect upon and evaluate practice for the evidence-based OT.

The type of research questions asked in phenomenological research might include:

- What is the meaning of independence for a disabled person? (e.g. McCuaig & Frank, 1991)
- What is the meaning of rehabilitation for patients following a cardiovascular accident (CVA)?

Box 5.3

Examples of OT phenomenological research include:

- Helm and Dickerson's (1995) study of a patient with a Colles' fracture. This research explored the patient's understanding of the effect of disability and the role of OT in the recovery of function. The key themes to emerge were the frustrations caused by the impairment of function and the patient's dissatisfaction with being given a 'standard' rehabilitation package. This research provides useful insights both into the experience of impairment and disability and patients' responses to rehabilitation interventions.
- Finlay's (1997) insightful study of how OTs view their clients. This research revealed how OTs use social evaluations and how clients can be categorised as 'good', 'bad', or 'difficult'.
- Whiteford's (1998) study exploring the development of OT students' understanding of cultural issues. She looked at the meanings students attribute to, and their understanding of, their experiences of working with people from different cultural groups and their perceptions of cultural differences.

The final qualitative approach to be discussed here is *grounded theory*. The main aim of grounded theory is theory-generation; a broad topic area is developed, the researcher then gathers data relevant to the topic using participants who might be seen to have a particular knowledge of the topic. The process of data collection is continued until the researcher feels all possible avenues are exhausted. Much of the early clinical reasoning research in OT adopted a grounded theory approach (Mattingly & Fleming, 1994).

Research methods in qualitative research

A variety of *methods* of data collection are used in qualitative research. The three main methods are:

- Interviews
- Observations
- Written materials

Box 5:4

Munroe (1996) used a combination of interviews and observations in her study of clinical reasoning in community OTs.

Whiteford (1998) used a series of interviews, over a 3-year period, to gather data on OT students' developing understanding of cultural diversity.

Finlay (1997) used interviews, with supporting data from her reflective field diary, to gather data on OTs' social evaluations of their clients.

Helm and Dickerson (1995) used a series of videotaped interviews to gather data on how their patient coped with her injury (Colles' fracture) and recovery.

Analysis, within qualitative research, is an ongoing process, which takes place throughout the research. Unlike quantitative research, where analysis takes place once data collection is completed, qualitative analysis consists of coding, describing and categorising the themes which emerge from the research data. A vital tool in this process is the researcher's field log and reflective diary (DePoy & Gitlin, 1994).

What makes 'good' qualitative research?

One of the problems to have bedevilled qualitative research is the issue of whether qualitative research can be seen as 'good' rigorous research. Frequently qualitative research is evaluated using criteria of validity and reliability, criteria that are suitable for quantitative research. However, criteria which focus on the generalisability or replicability of research are inappropriate for a methodology which seeks to describe experiences and social complexities (Krefting, 1991). This does not mean that qualitative research cannot be evaluated. It means, however, that a different approach must be used. It is important for evidence-based OTs to understand the ways of ensuring that qualitative research is rigorous in order to be able to appraise qualitative research from an appropriate perspective.

Trustworthiness in qualitative research

Krefting (1991) proposed that the notion of trustworthiness should be used when evaluating qualitative research. There are four aspects to trustworthiness and various strategies which qualitative researchers will use to ensure that their research is rigorous. Table 5.2 summarises the aspects and strategies of trustworthiness. The key components of each aspect will be outlined below, with examples from the OT research.

Table 5.2 Key aspects and strategies of trustworthiness.

Aspect	Strategy
Credibility	Prolonged and varied field experience Reflection and field diary Triangulation Member checking
Transferability	Nominated sample Comparison of sample with demographic data Dense description of the research setting
Dependability	Audit Triangulation Peer examination
Confirmability	Audit Triangulation Reflection

Credibility

The credibility of the research assesses whether the research is giving a true picture of the phenomenon being studied, based not on the researcher's expectations and assumptions but on the reality of the participants' experiences. A good test of credibility is whether the descriptions and interpretations of the phenomenon are recognisable to people outside the research setting.

There are various ways of ensuring credibility. To be able to get a true and detailed picture it is necessary to collect data over a prolonged period of time and from a range of participants. If possible, data should also be collected using a variety of research methods.

This process is known as triangulation. However, the length of time and the closeness of contact with participants can result in researchers finding it difficult to differentiate their own experiences from those of their participants. This is where a reflective approach (Finlay, 1998) is vitally important. The researcher should keep a field diary to enable reflexivity and to keep a record of thoughts, feelings, ideas and assumptions as the research progresses. A final strategy for ensuring credibility is to involve participants in the analysis of the research, by giving them access not only to the transcribed data but also to the interpretations and allowing them to comment on the research.

Box 5:5

Munroe (1996) ensured credibility in her research by triangulation and member checking. She used both observation and interviews to collect data. The observation data were given to each participant and used within the interview to explore clinical reasoning.

Whiteford (1998) used prolonged field experiences, gathering data over a 3-year period, in her study of OT students. She also used participant reflexivity and a field log as strategies to triangulate and ensure the credibility of her research.

Finlay's (1997) main credibility strategy was reflexivity in her study of OTs' social evaluations of their clients. Some member checking was done by two of the participants.

Helm and Dickerson's (1995) study of the experiences of hand injury appears to have used limited strategies to ensure credibility. However, within the limits of a small study, they did endeavour to achieve prolonged field experience by interviewing their participant on three occasions over the course of her treatment and rehabilitation.

Transferability

The second aspect of trustworthiness is whether the research can be seen as transferable to other settings. This can be seen in terms of how well the study achieves 'goodness of fit' with other contexts. Although, as Lincoln and Guba (1985) note, transferability is more the responsibility of the reader than the researcher. The researcher's task is to describe the setting in sufficient detail to allow comparisons to be drawn.

The strategies used to ensure transferability focus mainly on the sampling of participants for the study. The key factor is that the participants are a true representation of the group being studied. This can be done by attempting to match the participants to the demographic variables within the group as a whole, or by using a nominated sample. Nominated sampling is when key informants from the study group identify other people who could be seen as typical of the group.

Transferability can also be reviewed in terms of the denseness and detail given on the background information about the participants and the study group. This then allows the reader to assess the goodness of fit to other similar settings.

Box 5:6

Munroe (1996) established clear criteria for choosing participants for her study of community OTs. She also adopted a 'networking' approach to sampling to ensure representation of rural, urban and suburban OT services within her study.

Whiteford (1998) gave no details of her sampling procedures beyond stating that it was 'purposive'. The reader is left to assume that OT students in New Zealand are much like OT students anywhere else in the world.

Finlay's (1997) small sample of nine OTs were identified as a 'convenience' sample. However, from the brief description given her sample does appear to encompass a range of OT work settings.

Although Helm and Dickerson's (1995) study has only one participant, transferability can be assessed from the dense description given of the setting of the study.

Dependability

The dependability of a qualitative study relates to how consistent the data and findings are. In other words, in quantitative terms, how reliable the research is. However, as qualitative research cannot be subject to the same controls as quantitative research, the qualitative researcher can only ensure dependability by clearly explaining the process of the research. This allows the research to be audited and peer reviewed. The researcher should enlist the help of colleagues to review the research process.

> **Box 5:7**
>
> Peer evaluation and audit are mentioned by both Finlay (1997) and Whiteford (1998) as strategies used to ensure dependability in their research.

Confirmability

Confirmability refers to the strategies used by the researcher to limit bias within the research. In qualitative research this involves the neutrality, not of the researcher, but of the data. The researcher in qualitative research cannot remain outside the research situation. However, the neutrality of the data can be ensured by being reflective and keeping a detailed log of thoughts, ideas and assumption. The researcher can ask a colleague to audit the research and follow through the decision and analysis process. The researcher can also check ideas and interpretations with participants and expert colleagues.

> **Box 5:8**
>
> Munroe (1996) used member checking and expert review to ensure the confirmability of her results. She used focus group interviews with OTs to confirm her findings.
>
> Whiteford (1998) used reflexivity and audit to ensure confirmability in her study.
>
> Finlay (1997) used a number of strategies to ensure the confirmability of her findings. These included audit, member checking and reflexivity.

Appraising qualitative research

As with any appraisal, the appraisal of a qualitative study addresses three main questions:

- Are the results trustworthy?
- What are the results?
- How will these results help me work with my clients?

Table 5.3 gives an overview of the questions to ask when appraising a qualitative study. These questions are drawn from a range of sources including Krefting (1991), Gray (1997) and Greenhalgh (1997) and the author's own experience as a qualitative researcher.

Table 5.3 Questions to ask when critically appraising a qualitative study.

Are the results trustworthy?

- Was the research question clearly identified?
- Was a qualitative methodology and approach appropriate?
- Was the setting in which the research took place clearly described?
- Were the sampling processes planned, and clearly described?
- Was the data collection process clearly described?
- What methods were used to analyse the data?
- Were methods used to ensure the credibility of the research?
- Did the research workers address issues of confirmability and dependability?
- Were ethical issues considered?

What are the results?

- What were the key findings?
- Were the results presented in sufficient detail to assess the interpretation of the findings?
- Were the results of the research kept separate from the conclusions drawn by the research workers?
- If quantitative methods were appropriate, as a supplement to the qualitative methods, were they used?

How will these results help me work with my clients?

- Can the results be applied to my client group and interventions?

The reader will note that there are similarities in the questions asked to appraise any piece of research, be it a RCT, a qualitative study or a systematic review. The various questions will now be expanded, within the context of appraising a qualitative study. Table 5.4 gives a worked example of a critical appraisal of a qualitative study (Munroe, 1996).

Table 5.4 Worked example of a critical appraisal of a qualitative study using: Munroe, H. (1996) Clinical reasoning in community occupational therapy. *British Journal of Occupational Therapy*, **59**(5), 196–202.

Question	Yes/no/ can't tell	Comments
Are the results trustworthy?		
Was the research question clearly identified?	Yes	The focus of the study was clinical reasoning, and within that broad focus the aims and objectives of the study were clearly defined: The aim was to document and describe the nature and scope of clinical reasoning in community OT.
Was a qualitative methodology and approach appropriate?	Yes	The study aimed to describe the nature of clinical reasoning amongst a group of community OTs. This could only be achieved by exploring the participants' definitions and experience of clinical reasoning, for which qualitative methodology and a phenomenological approach are the most appropriate.
Was the setting in which the research took place clearly described?	No	The research stated that the respondents were all community OTs. However, this is the extent of the information given; it is not possible to assess the research's transferability in anything but general terms.

Contd

Table 5.4 *Contd.*

Question	Yes/no/ can't tell	Comments
If the answer to these screening questions is 'yes', is it worth carrying on with the appraisal?	Yes	With two 'yes' and one 'no' it seems appropriate to continue to appraise this research.
Were the sampling processes planned, and clearly described?	Yes/no	This could be a matter of some debate.To a greater extent there appears to be insufficient information to answer this question. The sampling process is described as purposive and certain criteria were established; attempts were made to ensure that the sample covered urban, suburban and rural OT services. However, the nature of the sampling process is not described in sufficient detail.
Was the data collection process clearly described?	Yes	The primary data collection methods were interview and observation. The researcher also kept a field diary. The process is adequately described and gives the reader a clear overview of the research process.
What methods were used to analyse the data?	—	Data analysis consisted of coding, classification and the development of concepts. These appear to be appropriate and adequate for the study.
Were methods used to ensure the credibility of the research?	Yes	There is evidence of triangulation (data collection by interview, observation and field diary), member checking (participants reviewed the coding and classification of the findings) and lengthy field experience (participants were observed and interviewed on a number of occasions).

Contd

Table 5.4 *Contd.*

Question	Yes/no/ can't tell	Comments
Did the research workers address issues of confirmability and dependability?	Yes	The findings were discussed both with the participants and with an expert group of clinicians (as part of a focus group). The researcher appears to have taken adequate measures to ensure confirmability and dependability.
Were ethical issues considered?	Can't tell	Issues of access, consent and confidentiality are not discussed in the paper.
What are the results?		
What were the key findings?	—	Three patterns of reasoning emerged from the study: • Reflexivity–reasoning–decision making • Reflexivity–decision making–reasoning • Decision making–reflexivity–reasoning. Three types of decisions were classified: • Technical • Procedural • Interactive
Were the results presented in sufficient detail to assess the interpretation of the findings?	No	The findings are summarised in the paper, but no attempt is made to explore each of the reasoning processes or classification of decisions. No examples of interview data. Therefore, whilst the findings are interesting they are of limited value as evidence as the detail is somewhat limited and the rigour of the findings cannot be adequately appraised.
Were the results of the research kept separate from the conclussions drawn by the research workers?	Yes	There is a clear division between the findings and the discussion and conclusion sections.

Contd

Table 5.4 *Contd.*

Question	Yes/no/ can't tell	Comments
If quantitative methods were appropriate, as a supplement to the qualitative methods, were they used?	Yes	Demographic data about the respondents and the types of observed visits are presented in table format. The frequency of the decisions taken by the category of decision is given. The quantitative data provided a useful supplement to the rather brief overview of the findings.
How will these results help me work with my clients?		*The answers to this question can only, really, be given by you, the reader, in relation to your service. These are my (the author's) reflections only.*
Can the results be applied to my client group and interventions?	Yes	The findings of the study support existing clinical reasoning literature and provide some information on the reasoning process of a small group of community OTs The paper provides useful 'food-for-thought' to any OT considering the thinking and clinical reasoning processes and as such can be seen as useful evidence for reflexivity-in-action and reflexivity-on-action (Schön, 1983).

Are the results trustworthy?

Was the research question clearly identified?

Although the research question in a qualitative study may be very broad, it is still important for the researchers to outline the aims and objectives of their study, to state a research question, and to give some idea about the parameters of the study.

Was a qualitative methodology and approach appropriate?

What was the study aiming to do? If the focus of the study was an exploration of a phenomenon or to gain an insight into particular issues, then a qualitative methodology is appropriate. Has the researcher identified the research approach used, i.e. ethnography, phenomenology, etc.? Is it the most appropriate approach?

Was the setting in which the research took place clearly described?

In terms of the transferability of the study, this is vitally important. The aim of the researcher should be to give the reader sufficient detail about the research setting for the reader to assess the goodness of fit with his or her own practice setting.

These questions can be used as a screening process to help you to decide whether it is worth spending precious reading time on a particular study. If the answers to these questions are negative it is probably not worth continuing to read and appraise the study, as it will provide poor-quality evidence of effectiveness or for reflexivity.

Were the sampling processes planned, and clearly described?

Is the sampling process clearly explained and justified? Did the researcher attempt to make the sample 'representative', either by matching demographic variables or by using a nominated sample? Sampling in qualitative studies can be difficult and researchers often have to resort to convenience or snowball sampling techniques. The researcher might have used the first x (number) people encountered who roughly fitted the study, and this might lead to a biased and unrepresentative sample.

Was the data collection process clearly described?

Data collection in qualitative research is often a long, complex and varied process. Have you been given enough information about what the researchers did, and why they chose to do the things they did? If observation was used, was the researcher an active or a passive participant in the setting? If interviews were used, has the researcher given you an overview of the themes and questions? How were the interviews recorded and transcribed? Did the researcher keep a field diary?

What methods were used to analyse the data?

Unlike statistical analysis, the analysis of qualitative data is time-consuming, complex, varied and does not have a standard format. However, has the researcher been systematic in the analysis? You should look out for details of how the data were coded. Is there evidence of *content analysis*, or a *constant comparative* approach? Did the researcher *immerse* him/herself in the data (DePoy & Gitlin, 1994)?

Were methods used to ensure the credibility of the research?

The strategies for ensuring credibility, discussed above, are prolonged field experience, triangulation, member checking and reflexivity. What evidence is there of these strategies being used in the research?

Did the research workers address issues of confirmability and dependability?

Was the research process subjected to audit by colleagues of the researcher? Is there sufficient detail in the report to allow you to audit the research? Were the participants involved in reviewing the interpretation of the data? An important aspect of any research is the data that do not fit neatly into the main themes of the analysis. How has the researcher dealt with this type of data?

Were ethical issues considered?

By its very nature, qualitative research can be an ethical minefield. Have ethical issues, such as access to participants, procedures for giving informed consent, the confidentiality and anonymity of information and participants, dealing with sensitive issues, the conflict of being a therapist/researcher, been addressed?

What are the results?

What were the key findings?

Results will be presented in terms of themes. Are the themes logical? Are they clearly explained? Do they reflect the aims of the study?

Were the results presented in sufficient detail to assess the interpretation of the findings?

It is important to review how the results were presented. The data of qualitative research are words. The results should include samples of the participants' actual words, rather than summaries of what was said. Where participants are quoted, they should also be identified in some way. Make sure that the full spread of participants has been quoted, not just one or two people who happened to say what the researcher wanted to hear.

Were the results of the research kept separate from the conclusions drawn by the research workers?

Quantitative research is presented in a standard format of Introduction, Methods, Results and Discussion. It is clear in any quantitative report what the findings (Results) were and how the researcher has interpreted them (Discussion). In qualitative research the results and discussion are often presented together. It is important, therefore, to assess how well the data and the interpretation are linked, and whether the interpretation seems logical.

If quantitative methods were appropriate, as a supplement to the qualitative methods, were they used?

Whilst statistical analysis is rarely appropriate within a purely qualitative study, it might be appropriate to present some findings in table format or in terms of quantitative data.

How will these results help me work with my clients?

Can the results be applied to my client group and interventions?

This question returns to the earlier question of transferability. If the goodness of fit is limited, the research might still give food for thought and evidence for reflexivity.

As Greenhalgh (1997) points out, as qualitative research is becoming more popular and more acceptable there is a danger that poor-quality qualitative research will be published. This is especially true as the tools for evaluating and appraising qualitative research are still being developed. However, as this chapter has shown, qualitative research can be rigorous and it can be appraised. With its focus on the insider perspective, qualitative research should provide the evidence-based OT with valuable evidence with which to explore the value and effectiveness of client-centred interventions.

Activity

- Identify a qualitative study of relevance to your area of practice/ interest
- Using the appraisal questions above, work with a colleague to appraise the article and to assess its value as evidence

Further reading

The following references will allow the reader to explore issues pertinent to the design and appraisal of qualitative research in more depth.

Bailey, D.M. (1997) *Research for the Health Professional*, 2nd edn. Philadelphia: FA Davis Co.

Burgess, R (1984) *In the Field*. London: Unwin Hyman.

Denzin, N.K. & Lincoln, Y.S. (eds) (1994) *Handbook of Qualitative Research*. Thousand Oaks: Sage.

DePoy, E. & Gitlin, L.N. (1994) *Introduction to Research*. St Louis: Mosby.

Grbich, C. (1999). *Qualitative Research in Health*. London: Sage.

Greenhalgh, T. (1997) *How to Read a Paper*. London: BMJ Publishing Group.

Kielhofner, G. (1982) Qualitative research: part two, methodological approaches and relevance to occupational therapy. *Occupational Therapy Journal of Research*, **2**, 150–70.

Krefting, L. (1991) Rigor in qualitative research: the assessment of trustworthiness. *American Journal of Occupational Therapy*, **45**(3), 214-22.

Popay, J., Rogers, A. & Williams, G. (1998) Rationale and standards for the systematic review of qualitative literature in health services research. *Journal of Qualitative Health Research*, **8**, 341-51.

Popay, J. & Williams, G. (1998) Qualitative research and evidence-based healthcare. *Journal of the Royal Society of Medicine*, **91**(Suppl. 35), 32-7.

Streubert, H.J. & Carpenter, D.R. (1995) *Qualitative Research in Nursing*. Philadelphia: JB Lippincott Co.

Yerxa, E.J (1991). Seeking a relevant, ethical, and realistic way of knowing for occupational therapy. *American Journal of Occupational Therapy*, **45**(3), 199–204.

Chapter 6
MAKING EVIDENCE-BASED PRACTICE WORK

The importance of clinical effectiveness and evidence-based practice are emphasised in government policy (NHS Executive, 1996; Walshe, 1998). The creation of a National Institute for Clinical Excellence (NICE), with its emphasis on evaluating the effectiveness of health care interventions both in terms of cost and clinical effectiveness, supports this policy (Department of Health, 1997). However, as Newell (1997) stated, much of the impetus for clinical effectiveness and evidence-based practice is focused at institutional levels. Others (e.g. Bury, 1998; Keep, 1998; Needham & Oliver, 1998) have written about the management, and management of change, aspects of making evidence-based health care work. The focus of this book has been much more practical. This chapter will, therefore, concentrate on practical ways in which OTs can become involved in evidence-based practice by using reflection, supervision and mentoring, through journal clubs, using and developing intervention guidelines and evidence-based audit of existing practice. However, the perceived barriers to evidence-based practice must be acknowledged and the chapter will conclude by looking at ways of identifying and overcoming the barriers to evidence-based OT and establishing an evidence-based climate for OT practice.

Using evidence-based practice in the practice/intervention setting

All OTs have an ethical responsibility to be:

> 'personally responsible for actively maintaining and developing their personal and professional competence and [to] base service delivery on accurate and current information in the interests of high quality care' (College of Occupational Therapists, 1995: para 5.4).

This emphasis on continuing professional development will be reinforced by the review of the Professions Supplementary to Medicine Act. Occupational therapists also have an ethical responsibility to:

> 'ensure that wherever possible their professional practice is based upon established research findings' (College of Occupational Therapists, 1995: para 5.6.3).

This places the onus on all practitioners to become evidence-based OTs. However, as we have seen, the potential sources of research evidence pertinent to OT are large. The average OT has little hope of managing to read *everything* pertinent to his or her field of practice.

Using reflection, supervision and mentoring to become an evidence-based OT

Many therapists wonder how to become involved in evidence-based practice without realising that they are already working within an evidence-based perspective. The processes of reflection, supervision and discussion with a mentor are all opportunities to review one's practice from an evidence-based perspective. Evidence-based practice, as we have seen, is not about *doing* research, it is about *using* research very explicitly to underpin the intervention decisions we make on a daily basis as practitioners.

As OTs we are encouraged to be reflective practitioners, to look critically at what we do. The process of reflection involves describing an event and then looking at the decision-making and reasoning process which underpin the actions taken within that event. The event concerned can be any interaction with a client. These reflections can form the basis of supervision or mentoring discussions.

To make the reflective process evidence-based it is necessary to address the following questions:

- Is there any evidence to underpin the intervention decisions I made in this situation?
- Have I searched for the evidence to underpin this intervention?
- Am I using evidence to underpin the decisions I made in this situation?
- Have I critically appraised this evidence?
- Are there any professional or local standards and guidelines that are relevant to this intervention and situation?
- Have I critically appraised this information?
- Am I involving the client in the decisions about intervention?
- Am I informing the client of the evidence-base for these interventions?
- Am I regularly updating my knowledge?
- Am I sharing and disseminating the evidence I have gathered?

Reflective and evidence-based practice should not be threatening. By thinking through and articulating the reasoning processes we use, unconsciously, every day we can strengthen, rather than weaken, our practice. Outdated and redundant interventions can be stopped and effective interventions can be reinforced.

Student OTs on fieldwork placements can be a useful aid to the evidence-based OT. Students are encouraged to be reflective and they are encouraged to question and explore the clinical reasoning processes they are using. They also have search and research skills and access to their university libraries. As part of their reflections on the interventions they are involved with, students should be encouraged to search for and present the evidence to underpin the interventions.

Journal clubs

One way of ensuring focused reading, and to develop an evidence-based climate, is to establish a *journal club*. Journal clubs are groups of people (from three to ten members) who meet regularly (every one or two months) to review and discuss one or more articles of relevance to their practice. Journal clubs can provide useful opportunities to practise the critical appraisal skills discussed in the previous chapters. Membership of, and commitment to, a journal club could provide useful evidence of continuing professional development for an individual's professional portfolio and appraisal.

Journal clubs have been a part of medical practice for many years (Linzer, 1987). These journal clubs often consisted of one person presenting a critical review of an article to colleagues. However, as Sackett *et al*. (1997) pointed out, this type of journal club is becoming extinct. A much more successful, and useful, format for journal clubs, advocated by Linzer *et al*. (1988) and Sackett *et al*. (1997), is a journal club based on a critical appraisal format. Here a group of colleagues meet together to share a discussion and appraisal of one of more papers, probably using an appraisal checklist (see previous chapters) as a way of structuring the discussion.

Journal clubs, using an appraisal format, not only provide a forum for practising appraisal skills, but can also provide an opportunity to review and reflect upon current practice. The outcome of a journal club discussion may be to implement changes to current interventions or practice. The journal club has provided a valuable opportunity for colleagues to explore issues, share ideas, consider differing perspectives and participate in the shaping and developing of departmental practice and policy. Box 6.1 gives an overview and format for establishing a journal club.

Box 6:1

Planning

For a journal club to run well, it needs to be planned and organised, and members should be committed to the success of the group.

- Leadership – the journal club needs an overall convenor who will lead and plan meetings, although each meeting can be led by different members of the group.
- Membership – the size of the group should be from three to ten people who are committed to the idea of the journal club.

- Establish regular meetings – set a timetable and plan meetings in advance, decide on a regular time and day for the meetings.
- Find a location – identify a suitable, informal, location where the club can meet with minimal interruptions. The meeting could be combined with lunch.
- Decide on the themes to be discussed – this might take place at the first meeting of the group. Decide on clear evidence-based questions with clearly identified problems, interventions and outcomes. Decide who will be responsible for organising and running each session.
- Liaise with the librarian – having established the themes/evidence-based questions, each session leader will need to find relevant articles for the group to discuss. Work with your librarians to find the articles.
- Distribute/photocopy articles – make sure that all members of the group have access to copies of the articles for discussion at least a week before the meeting.

The meeting

- Use an appraisal checklist (see previous chapters).
- Set clear time limits – spend the majority of the session discussing the chosen article(s), but allow time at the end of the session to discuss the implications for your department and to make an action plan if changes are to be made.
- Avoid 'critical appraisal nihilism' (Sackett *et al.*, 1997: 193) – all research has flaws, but most research can be useful.
- Don't get 'tied up' on the numbers – focus on the key outcomes rather than whether a *t*-test really was the best analysis.
- Make sure that everyone has a chance to join in.
- Establish an 'open' climate, where any contribution is accepted and valued.
- Have fun and enjoy the discussions.

Follow-up

- Make sure that any action plans, reflections, ideas for change are referred to the appropriate people.
- Keep notes of the topics discussed and the outcomes.

Journal clubs can be uni-professional or multi-disciplinary. It will depend on your setting which is the most appropriate. Each meeting can look at single articles or a number of articles. Single articles can be useful to start with as everyone develops their appraisal skills. However, although looking at a number of papers may take longer, it will give a broader and more interesting perspective on any given topic or evidence-based question.

Journal clubs do require time and an element of commitment. Given the current climate of clinical effectiveness and continuing professional development, managers should encourage and facilitate the establishment of journal clubs. Searching for relevant articles may feel like an onerous responsibility, but if searching and session leadership is divided among the group members it should not prove a too difficult and time-consuming task.

Activity

Establish a journal club:

- Collect together a group of like-minded colleagues
- Establish a time for regular meetings
- Decide on a number of evidence-based questions and allocate the planning of each session
- Meet as a journal club

Evidence-based audit

Another approach all OTs can use to incorporate evidence into their practice is through evidence-based audit. Audit has been part of National Health Service (NHS) policy for medicine, nursing and profession allied to medicine (PAMS) throughout the 1990s (Department of Health, 1991), and can be defined as:

> 'The systematic critical appraisal of the quality of clinical care including the procedures for diagnosis, treatment and care, the associated use of resources and the resulting outcome and quality of life for the patient' (NHS Management Executive, 1994).

The systematic process of audit has involved establishing standards and protocols for intervention and care and then using these standards and protocols to review the quality of care received by clients. They have rarely been based on evidence.The focus of audit has been on enhancing and improving the *quality* of health and social care. However, the current climate of health and social care focuses on *clinical effectiveness* (NHS Executive, 1996). This has placed the emphasis on the synthesis of audit and evidence-based practice, resulting in the development of the process of *evidence-based audit*. Table 6.1 summarises the similarities and differences between audit and evidence-based audit.

Table 6.1 Comparison of audit and evidence-based audit.

Audit	Evidence-based audit
Identify clinical audit topic	Identify clinical audit topic Find relevant research evidence and expert information Critically appraise the evidence
Agree standards, protocols and guidelines	Agree evidence-based standards, protocols and guidelines
Implement standards, protocols	Implement evidence-based standards, protocols, guidelines
Assess compliance with standards, protocols and guidelines	Assess compliance with evidence-based standards, protocols and guidelines
Review standards, protocols and guidelines	Review evidence-based standards, protocols and guidelines (this will involve finding and appraising any new evidence)
Agree changes (if required)	Agree changes (if required)
Implement reviewed and refined standards, protocols and guidelines	Implement reviewed and refined standards, protocols and guidelines

The focus of audit has been to set standards and guidelines based on local knowledge and expertise. The focus of evidence-based audit is to add research evidence to the expertise and experience of local practitioners. The process of developing and auditing clinical (or intervention) guidelines will be discussed in the next section. It is not the function of this book to give a step-by-step account of the evidence-based audit process. Rather the aim of this book is to highlight how the reader can become an evidence-based OT and to highlight the resources available for evidence-based OTs to develop their skills. Numerous books and articles have been published on the process of audit and evidence-based audit, including Arnold *et al.* (1995), Kogan *et al.* (1995), Malby (1995) and Buttery (1998). All NHS Trusts should have clinical effectiveness and/or clinical audit departments who will be able to help in the development of evidence-based audit of local OT services. Evidence-based audit should not be a solitary task, although it can be used as a process for reflecting upon and reviewing your own practice. A much better approach to evidence-based audit is for a group of colleagues, within one intervention setting, to work together to review, reflect upon and audit their interventions and practice. The process of evidence-based audit might lead to the development of local guidelines for practice and interventions.

Activity

- Meet with a number of colleagues to reflect on practice and to develop topics for evidence-based audit
- Identify and locate the clinical effectiveness/audit personnel within your NHS Trust or service setting
- Discuss the topics for evidence-based audit with the clinical effectiveness/audit personnel
- Establish an audit strategy for your setting

Clinical guidelines

Guidelines for practice have been developed over recent years. These guidelines aim to improve, focus and direct intervention and practice. Guidelines have been used to underpin good practice and are often used as tools within the audit process (see previous section). Guidelines have been developed at local (Moreton, 1998) and national (College of Occupational Therapists, 1990; Canadian Association of Occupational Therapists, 1991; American Occupational Therapy Association, 1996; Canadian Association of Occupational Therapists, 1997) level.

Clinical guidelines have been defined as:

> 'Systematically developed statements to assist practitioner decisions about appropriate health care for specific clinical circumstances' (Thomas *et al.*, 1999: 2).

They are seen as tools to help managers and practitioners decide about the process of intervention. Guidelines provide principles upon which to base interventions and service delivery, and against which the standards and quality of interventions and service delivery can be assessed and measured. Austin and Herbert (1995) outlined the purpose of clinical guidelines as:

- Collecting sound evidence of the efficacy of a pattern of behaviour, for example randomised controlled trials (RCTs)
- Providing expert knowledge in an agreed and easy-to-use format
- Making knowledge accessible to therapists when they need it
- Supporting intervention decision making
- Supporting care plan negotiation between client and therapist
- Raising the standards of care
- Supporting management functions, especially contracting and budgeting

The goal of any guideline is to improve the quality of health and social care. An excellent example of a guideline which has been instrumental in improving the delivery and quality of OT practice is the work done in Canada developing client-centred practice in OT (Canadian Association of Occupational Therapists, 1991, 1997; Law, 1998).

However, these guidelines have rarely been evidence-based. They have been drawn from a synthesis of current best practice, consensus views of practitioners and expert discussion. With the current emphasis on evidence-based health and social care, there is a need to develop more rigorous, systematic and evidence-based guidelines (Mann, 1996). These *clinical guidelines* need to be based on current best evidence of effectiveness. Only where evidence is of poor quality, or absent, should expert and professional opinion be used as evidence. These guidelines should focus on specific interventions with specific client groups, much as the evidence-based questions discussed in Chapter 1 have a specific problem, intervention and outcome focus. Clinical guidelines should be based, if possible, on systematic reviews of the relevant evidence. Where clinical guidelines differ from systematic reviews is that a clinical guideline will develop and outline clear recommendations and principles upon which practice and interventions can be based. Systematic reviews give both the statistical and clinical significance of the findings, but do not attempt to go beyond these or make recommendations about the interventions.

Clinical guidelines can be used as the tools to improve and change practice. Examples of how guidelines and evidence have been used in this way include the development of 'integrated care pathways' for stroke patients (Dunning *et al.*, 1998). Clinical guidelines can be seen as the end-product of an evidence-based approach, where evidence is reviewed and synthesised to improve intervention and OT practice not only for an individual client but also for a group of clients with a particular problem or need. However, there appears to be no evidence of the use of clinical guidelines within OT (Thomas, 1999), and few examples of evidence-based clinical guidelines relevant to OT. Austin and Herbert (1995) sought to stimulate debate amongst OTs about the development, value and use of clinical guidelines. However, little debate appears to have been forthcoming.

Box 6.2

An example of a set of evidence-based clinical guidelines which is being used by OTs is the *Guidelines for the collaborative rehabilitative management of elderly people who have fallen* (Occupational Therapy for Elderly People (OCTEP), 1997; Simpson *et al.*, 1998).

These guidelines have been designed specifically for OTs and physiotherapists working with older people who have fallen. The guidelines outline the aims of intervention with this group of clients as:

- Improving ability to withstand threats to balance
- Improving the safety of the environment
- Preventing the consequences of a long lie on the floor
- Optimising confidence in their ability to move safely

Assessment and intervention guidelines are given.

A national audit of the dissemination and use of these guidelines is currently being undertaken.

Sackett *et al.* (1997:50) proposed a single appraisal question for any guideline:

> 'does this guideline offer an opportunity for significant improvement in the quality of health care practice?'

The process of implementing the principles outlined within a clinical guideline will require not only individual but institutional commitment to change. A team approach is necessary as guidelines are unlikely to affect the practice of only one professional group. Management support is required and a formal system of review must be established to audit the effectiveness of, and the effect of implementation, of the guideline.

One of the dilemmas for OTs thinking about adopting clinical guidelines is a potential conflict between a client-centred philosophy of practice and what might be seen as the rigidity of a clinical guideline. However, clinical guidelines are just that, they are *guidelines* for practice. Clinical guidelines are one of the tools available to the evidence-based OT and, remembering the definition of Sackett *et al.* (1997) for evidence-based practice as the *judicious* use of best evidence, so should be used judiciously as part of the negotiation of a care plan or intervention process with the client.

Activity

- Identify any existing clinical guidelines relevant to your area of intervention and practice
- Discuss the practicalities of implementing these guidelines with your manager
- Identify other professional groups who might be affected by the implementation of these guidelines
- Discuss the practicalities of implementing these guidelines with this multi-disciplinary team
- Establish a strategy for the implementation of the guidelines
- Establish clear outcomes to be used as measures to assess the impact of the implementation of the clinical guidelines
- Discuss an audit strategy with your local clinical audit/effectiveness department
- Implement the guidelines

Barriers to evidence-based practice

A growing body of evidence exists suggesting that OTs (and other PAMS colleagues) are not confident evidence-based practitioners (Turner & Whitefield, 1996, 1997; Brown, 1998; Wiles & Barnard, 1998; Upton, 1999a,b). Upton (1999a) found that OTs held very positive attitudes towards the value of evidence-based practice. However, they rated their evidence-based practice knowledge and skills as low, especially in terms of the technical skills of evidence-based practice. Upton (1999a) defined the technical skills of evidence-based practice as IT skills, literature searching skills and research skills. Both Turner and Whitefield (1996, 1997) and Wiles and Barnard (1998) found that physiotherapists, whilst accepting the need for evidence-based approaches to practice, tended to rely on personal experience, practice-related courses and personal knowledge when selecting interventions. Wiles and Barnard (1998) found that physiotherapists perceived potential conflicts between:

- Evidence-based practice and existing experiential knowledge
- Evidence-based practice and patient-orientated practice

- Evidence-based practice and the independent and autonomous status of practitioners

Sumsion (1997) has also highlighted the potential conflict between evidence-based practice and client-centred philosophies of practice.

The need for OTs to embrace evidence-based practice has also been recognised and encouraged with special issues of both the *British Journal of Occupational Therapy* (College of Occupational Therapists, 1997) and the *Canadian Journal of Occupational Therapy* (Canadian Association of Occupational Therapists, 1998) dedicated to evidence-based practice and conferences on evidence-based practice in mental health (*British Journal of Therapy & Rehabilitation*, 1996). However, a number of authors (e.g. Taylor, 1997; Clemence, 1998; Wilson-Barnett, 1998) have highlighted the potential conflict between the qualitative research methodologies favoured by nursing and the PAMS and the high status given to RCTs in evidence-based practice. This should present less of a problem in the future with the growing acceptance of qualitative research within evidence-based practice (Popay & Williams, 1998).

Whilst evidence-based practice and evidence of clinical effectiveness are the driving forces in current health and social care, there are a number of barriers to the utilisation of evidence-based practice by OTs. These barriers are summarised in Table 6.2.

Table 6.2 Barriers to evidence-based practice.

- Access to, and availability of, information
- Limited time
- Lack of evidence-based practice skills
- Confidence in the value of the evidence that is available
- Support from management and colleagues
- Conflict with the client-centred philosophy of OT

Upton's (1999b) research identified, in descending order of importance, the following factors that would increase the use of evidence-based approaches to practice:

- More time
- Better dissemination
- Greater library resources
- Money
- Greater availability of IT
- Greater commitment from management
- Better access to the Internet

The various barriers, highlighted in Table 6.2, can be overcome.

Access to, and availability of, information

Access to the relevant information can be seen in terms of having access to suitable library resources and also being able to find the relevant information in the vast array of journals available to the evidence-based OT. However, access may also be limited because of the lack of dissemination of research findings. Research evidence may only be available in the 'grey' (or unpublished) literature. Research findings may be presented at conferences but never make it into print. Published evidence might not be read. Anecdotal evidence suggests that although the 'Falls' guidelines were disseminated through articles both in the *British Journal of Occupational Therapy* (Simpson *et al.*, 1998) and the OCTEP newsletter (Occupational Therapy for Elderly People, 1997), not all OTs working with older clients are aware of the existence of these guidelines.

Limited time

Time, for most OTs, is frequently seen as a scarce commodity. However, time for evidence-based practice activity can be acknowledged, possibly through the appraisal system.

Lack of evidence-based practice skills

The key evidence-based practice skills which appear to be needed are:

- IT skills
- Literature searching skills
- Critical appraisal skills

The Critical Appraisal Skills Programme (CASP) workshops (see Chapter 7) can be used to address both searching and appraisal skills development. These skills can then be cascaded throughout a department.

Confidence in the value of the evidence that is available

There is a growing body of evidence (e.g. Wiles & Barnard, 1998; Upton, 1999b) that therapists are less willing to act on research evidence than they are to act on other forms of evidence to review or change their practice. Upton (1999b) found, in descending order of willingness to act, that therapists would act on information from the following sources:

- Own practice and experience
- Colleagues from the same profession
- Line manager
- Journal articles
- Clinical effectiveness facilitator
- Colleagues from different professions
- The Internet

when reviewing or changing their practice. From this evidence there would appear to be a mismatch between the accepted hierarchy of evidence for evidence-based practice and the value therapists place on various sources of evidence.

Support from management and colleagues

Establishing an evidence-based culture must come from both managers and practitioners. Journal clubs (see above) can be useful ways of beginning to develop an evidence-based culture within a department. The objectives set as part of the development and appraisal process can be used to underpin the development of an evidence-based culture by making the goals of finding, appraising and using evidence explicit, thus ensuring that time should be allocated to evidence-based activity.

Conflict with the client-centred philosophy of OT

If evidence-based practice is seen, as Sackett *et al.* (1997) proposed, as the judicious use of current best evidence, then there is no conflict between an evidence-based and a client-centred philosophy of practice. Upton (1999a,b) identified 'involving patients fully in their care' as a key component of evidence-based practice. This aspect of evidence-based practice was the component most frequently used by the therapists in Upton's research. Discussing the effectiveness of proposed interventions with any client can only enhance the client-centred philosophy of any OT's practice.

Brown (1998) proposed the following strategies as useful for practitioners wanting to become evidence-based OTs:

- Adopt a 'spirit of enquiry'
- Read widely and critically
- Attend professional conferences
- Become involved in a journal club
- Collaborate with a researcher
- Develop strategic alliances

For the manager wishing to develop an evidence-based culture, the following strategies might be useful:

- Foster a climate of intellectual curiosity
- Offer emotional and moral support
- Offer resources and financial support
- Reward evidence-based initiatives and efforts
- Be a role model and a mentor

Activity

- Identify which of the barriers to becoming an evidence-based OT (outlined above) are most applicable to you and your work setting – a collaborative approach to this activity might be useful
- Outline the strategies most suitable to overcoming the barriers you have identified
- Discuss the barriers and strategies with your line manager
- Develop a strategy for becoming an evidence-based OT

The benefits of evidence-based practice have been outlined by Rosenberg and Donald (1995). These benefits are presented in Table 6.3. Whilst evidence-based practice is too new within occupational therapy to have been evaluated, there is evidence from medicine of its effectiveness (Bennett *et al.*, 1987; Shin *et al.*, 1993).

Table 6.3 Benefits of practising evidence-based health care.

For individual practitioners

- Enables practitioners to upgrade their knowledge-base routinely
- Improves practitioners' critical understanding of research methods and practice
- Improves confidence in management decisions
- Improves computer literacy and data searching skills
- Improves reading habits

For departments

- Gives a framework for group problem-solving and teaching
- Enables everyone to contribute to the team

For patients

- More effective use of resources
- Better communication with patients about the rationale behind intervention proposals

Further reading

The following references will give the reader more scope to explore the complexities of implementing evidence-based practice within OT and beyond.

Alnervik, A. & Svidén, G. (1996) On clinical reasoning: patterns of reflection on practice. *Occupational Therapy Journal of Research*, **16**(2), 98–110.

Castle, A. (1996) Developing an ethos of reflective practice for continuing professional development. *British Journal of Therapy and Rehabilitation*, **3**(7), 358–9.

Dunning, M., Abi-Aad, G., Gilbert, D., Gillam, S. & Livett, H. (1998) *Turning Evidence into Everyday Practice*. London: King's Fund.

Fish, D., Twinn, S., Purr, B. *et al.* (1991) *Promoting Reflection: Improving the Supervision of Practice Health Visiting and Initial Teacher Training*. London: West London Institute of Higher Education, West London Press.

Heasell, S. (1996) The risky economics of evidence-based medicine. *Health Care Risk Report*, November, 22–4.

Hicks, N.R. & Mant, J. (1997) Using the evidence: putting the research into practice. *British Journal of Midwifery*, **5**(7), 396–9.

Hunt, M. (1987) The process of translating research findings into nursing practice. *Journal of Advanced Nursing*, **12**, 101–10.

Landry, D.W. & Mathews, M. (1998) Economic evaluation of occupational therapy: where are we at? *Canadian Journal of Occupational Therapy*, **65**(3), 160–67.

Newdick, C. (1996) The status of guidelines. *Health Care Risk Report*, October, 14–15.

Schön, D. (1983) *The Reflective Practitioner*. New York: Basic.

Stewart, R. (1998) More art than science? *Health Service Journal*, 26 March, 28–9.

Walshe, K. (1996) Evidence-based health care – brave new world? *Health Care Risk Report*, March, 16–18.

Chapter 7
USEFUL RESOURCES

This chapter will provide the reader with an annotated list of sources of information and resources which may be helpful in the practice of evidence-based occupational therapy. These resources include:

- Indexes and databases
- Web sites
- E-mail discussion groups
- Further reading
  - Books
  - Evidence-based journals and publications
- Useful addresses and other miscellaneous resources

The author makes no apology for including a large number of resources which are Internet based. Whilst in 1997 it might have been appropriate to call Gray (1997) idealistic in proposing that every evidence-based practitioner should have not only access to a library and a supportive librarian but also access to:

- The Cochrane Library, MEDLINE, EMBASE and HealthSTAR
- The World Wide Web
- A personal computer with reference management software so that evidence can be stored systematically (Taylor, 1997)

access to the Internet is much more widespread today. With the government's current focus on information for health care and the development of an information strategy for the National Health

Service (NHS) (NHS Executive, 1998) it seems appropriate to include as much information as possible on Internet-based resources. The aim of the National Electronic Library for Health (NeLH) is:

- To provide easy access to best current knowledge
- To improve health and health care, clinical practice and patient choice

The target is to provide clinicians with access to information within 15 seconds. The aim is for NeLH to be in place and functioning by 2005.

Every effort has been made to ensure that the information presented here is as up to date as possible. However, the author cannot accept responsibility for errors but does apologise for any oversights! This resource information should be seen as a starting point and readers should annotate the text with their own additional resources, thus enabling each OT to build up a personal evidence-based practice resource.

Indexes and databases

In terms of the OT literature, the most comprehensive coverage can probably be found using a combination of AMED and CINAHL. However background material might be more easily found on ASSIA and MEDLINE. Access to databases is available via a variety of formats: hard copy, CD-ROM and the Internet. The tendency, currently, is for libraries to move away from subscriptions to hard copies and CD-ROM copies of databases and to move towards subscriptions via the Internet. Databases on CD-ROM use a variety of software, e.g. Ovid, SilverPlatter, which have slightly different search strategies. If possible, the evidence-based OT should access all databases through the same software as this makes transferring search skills rather easier. As was highlighted in Chapter 2, databases are only as good as their indexing and hand searching remains the most thorough and accurate search method.

AMED

AMED is the Allied and Alternative Medicine Database. It is produced by the British Library Health Care Information Service and contains bibliographic references from 1985 onwards. It covers the fields of complementary and allied medicine. The scope and coverage of the database is predominantly European with English as the most common language. The database includes references relevant to OT, physiotherapy, alternative medicine, palliative care, rehabilitation medicine and podiatry. The various topic areas were originally indexed separately (e.g. OT Index) but the indexes were amalgamated into AMED in 1998. AMED currently indexes around 400 journals, including the following OT journals:

American Journal of Occupational Therapy
Australian Occupational Therapy Journal
British Journal of Occupational Therapy
British Journal of Therapy and Rehabilitation
Canadian Journal of Occupational Therapy
Journal of Occupational Science – Australia
Occupational Therapy in Health Care
Occupational Therapy in Mental Health
Occupational Therapy Journal of Research
OT Practice
Physical and Occupational Therapy in Geriatrics
Physical and Occupational Therapy in Pediatrics
South African Journal of Occupational Therapy

The thesaurus uses a modified form of the MeSH (medical subject heading) headings. AMED is available on CD-ROM, in printed format and on the Internet. The separate indexes (OT Index, Physiotherapy Index, Rehabilitation Index, Palliative Care Index, Podiatry Index and Complementary Medicine) are also available in print format. The print versions of the indexes and AMED are available monthly.

More details are also available on:

http://www.silverplatter.com/catalog/amed.htm

Although AMED is an extremely useful resource for the evidence-based OT, it does appear to be somewhat 'selective' in its indexing. Articles which should be identified in a search are sometimes missed when searching AMED. All items included in AMED are available from the British Library Document Supply Centre. The British Library will carry out searches on AMED.

ASSIA

ASSIA is the Applied Social Sciences Index and Abstracts and is produced by Bowker-Saur. It is a key source for social science references, but has a good coverage of applied social care topics. Because it is UK produced, it has a good coverage of UK-based literature as well as literature from further afield. Of the journals included in ASSIA, five are OT journals. These OT-specific journals are:

American Journal of Occupational Therapy
Australian Occupational Therapy Journal
British Journal of Occupational Therapy
Occupational Therapy International
Scandinavian Journal of Occupational Therapy

ASSIA is available on-line and in both CD-ROM and print format, with quarterly CD and bi-monthly print updates.

BIDS

The Bath Information Data Service (BIDS) acts as a vehicle for subscription to a variety of citation indexes and other databases, including EMBASE and the British Education Index (see ERIC), through a password. This means that BIDS is only accessible through registered subscribers, such as universities. BIDS includes three Citation Indexes:

Scisearch (sciences)
Social Scisearch (social sciences)
Arts & Humanities Search

Citation Indexes are useful resources for searching forward in time, taking a particular reference and searching to find which authors have used that particular reference. For example, you might find a particular outcome measure and want to search for other literature where that measure has been used. Citation Indexes will allow you to input the name of the author of the outcome measure article and search for all uses of that article in published literature.

BIDS also contains IBSS (International Bibliography of the Social Sciences), which gives access to data from over 2600 international social science journals.

CINAHL

CINAHL is the Cumulated Index to Nursing and Allied Health Literature and is produced by CINAHL Information Systems in California. As its name suggests, it provides a database for nursing and allied literature. Like MEDLINE, CINAHL has a somewhat American bias. The majority of journals included in CINAHL have a nursing focus. However, some 43 therapy-related journals are included and of these 14 are specific to OT. The OT-specific journals include:

American Journal of Occupational Therapy
Australian Occupational Therapy Journal
British Journal of Occupational Therapy
Canadian Journal of Occupational Therapy
Journal of Occupational Science – Australia
New Zealand Journal of Occupational Therapy
Occupational Therapy in Health Care
Occupational Therapy in Mental Health
Occupational Therapy International
Occupational Therapy Journal of Research

OT Practice
Physical and Occupational Therapy in Geriatrics
Physical and Occupational Therapy in Pediatrics
Scandinavian Journal of Occupational Therapy

Other journals included in CINAHL, which might be of interest, include:

Activities, Adaptation and Aging
Assistive Technology
Therapy Weekly
WORK: A Journal of Prevention, Assessment and Rehabilitation

CINAHL uses a modified MeSH (medical subject heading) thesaurus. CINAHL is available in CD-ROM format, as a bi-monthly print up-date and on-line.

More details can be found at the CINAHL Web site at:

http://www.cinahl.com/

The Cochrane Library

The Cochrane Library is an electronic library 'designed to provide the evidence needed for healthcare decision making' (Gray, 1997: 222). The main focus of the Cochrane Library is to co-ordinate and collate the systematic review of evidence. The Cochrane Library is available on CD-ROM and on-line, and the CD-ROM is updated quarterly. It consists of a number of databases including:

- The Cochrane Database of Systematic Reviews
- The Cochrane Controlled Trials Register
- The York Database of Abstracts of Reviews of Effectiveness

Databases such as AMED, MEDLINE, etc., include articles because they have been published in the journals which the database includes in its listing. The merits of the article are based on the fact that the journal chose to publish it and that the database chose to include that journal in its listings. No attempt is made to exclude articles on the basis of their research type or because they are not research-based. The Cochrane Library is different. The Cochrane Library contains only research-based information. In fact, all of the information in the Cochrane Library is based on randomised controlled trials (RCTs) and controlled clinical trials (CCTs), which explains why the Cochrane Library might be seen as of limited value in the search for OT-relevant literature. However this is not the case as OT literature is being included in the Controlled Trials Register and OTs are involved with Systematic Review Groups.

The Cochrane Database of Systematic Reviews

Systematic reviews were discussed in detail in chapter 4. Throughout the world groups of researchers work together in Cochrane Collaboration Groups to collate and review the research evidence for specific health care interventions. The output from these groups, in the form of review protocols and completed reviews, are made available to a wider audience though the Cochrane Database of Systematic Reviews. Review groups of interest to OTs include:

Community mental health teams (CMHT) management of severe mental illness
Fall prevention in the elderly
Hip fracture: in-patient rehabilitation
Hospital at home
Life skills programmes for schizophrenia
Reality orientation (RO) for dementia
Reminiscence therapy (RT) for dementia

Abstracts of Cochrane reviews are available on the Web at both the UKCC (UK Cochrane Collaboration) site:

http://www.cochrane.co.uk/

and at the NHS CRD (NHS Centre for Reviews and Dissemination) Web site, as part of the-online version of the DARE database (see below for more information on DARE), at:

http://nhscrd.york.ac.uk/welcome.html

The Cochrane Collaboration now has a Physical Therapy and Rehabilitation Field which is co-ordinated through the University of Maastricht. This group can be contacted, via e-mail on:

hcw.devet@epid.rulimburg.nl

The Cochrane Controlled Trials Register

The aim of the Cochrane Controlled Trials Register is to index all RCTs and clinical trials, thus providing a comprehensive database for evidence-based practice. Trials are identified by volunteers hand searching relevant journals. OT specific journals are now being hand searched and included on the Register. This is a painstaking process. However, the Cochrane Controlled Trials Register does now include information pertinent to OTs.

A self-training guide to the Cochrane Library is available on the Web at:

http://libsun1.jr2.ox.ac.uk/a-ordd/index.htm

This training guide consists of a guide in Word 6.0, with accompanying PowerPoint files. The guide and these files can be downloaded from the Web site and can be copied or edited as required. However, readers should note that the authors of the guide give no commitment to keep this guide up to date. The guide does provide a useful overview of what to expect from the Cochrane Library, how to find information within the Cochrane Library and how to interpret the information.

Cochrane Library materials, including training materials, are available on the Centre for Reviews and Dissemination Web site, at:

http://www.york.ac.uk/inst/crd/cochlib.htm

The teaching and self-learning materials include comprehensive self-teaching guides to the Cochrane Library and systematic reviews, teaching materials (including PowerPoint slides, examples of evidence-based questions) and a short guide to the Cochrane Library. All of these materials can be downloaded, free of charge, from the Web site and can be adapted for individual teaching needs and uses.

DARE

Database of Abstracts of Reviews of Effectiveness (DARE) is produced by the NHS Centre for Reviews and Dissemination (NHS CRD) (see below). DARE provides a record of good-quality research-based reviews of the effectiveness of health care interventions, management and organisation. The staff at NHS CRD evaluate the reviews against quality criteria and provide abstracts of those reviews which meet the quality standards. This information can, therefore, be seen as being kite-marked for research quality. DARE also includes records of other useful reviews which do not meet the quality standards. DARE can be viewed as a source of overviews of high-quality reviews of evidence. However, because of its quantitative focus, DARE may be of limited value for many OTs.

DARE is available on disc, CD-ROM (as part of the Cochrane Library) and on-line at:

http://www.york.ac.uk/inst/cdr/dissem.htm

EMBASE

EMBASE is seen by many people as the European version of MEDLINE. It is produced in the Netherlands by Elsevier Science. As well as having a more European focus, it tends to focus on the more pharmacological aspects of medicine, although *Section 19: Physical Medicine and Rehabilitation* may be of use. EMBASE is available on CD-ROM (updated quarterly), in print format (updated bi-monthly) and as a series of topic-specific publications. EMBASE can also be accessed through BIDS (see above).

ERIC International

ERIC International contains a cluster of *education* databases, comprising British, Australian and Canadian Education Indexes.

The British Education Index contains bibliographic references to significant journal and thesis literature. With its education focus, this might be a useful database for OTs working with children in a range of settings.

MEDLINE

MEDLINE is the world's largest and most popular medical database. It is produced by the American National Library of Medicine (NLM). The printed version of the database was started in the 1870s by John Shaw Billings and is still produced as *Index Medicus*. The database was computerised in 1966 and became known as MEDLINE. MEDLINE is also available via the Internet as PubMed (see below). The journals included in MEDLINE are predominantly American peer-reviewed journals and, as the name suggests, the focus is on medical rather than related journals. Of the 3800 journals included in MEDLINE only one is an OT journal. The OT journal included is the *American Journal of Occupational Therapy*. However, other relevant journals which are of interest include:

Alternative Therapies in Health and Medicine
American Journal of Physical Medicine and Rehabilitation
International Journal of Rehabilitation Research

MEDLINE is available on CD-ROM and because of its popularity will be available in most medical libraries. Whilst MEDLINE might not be the first database to choose for an evidence-based OT, it will give access to some OT literature and to a reasonable range of background medical literature. The thesaurus uses the MeSH (medical subject heading) system.

NRR (National Research Register)

The National Research Register (NRR) is a register of on-going and recently completed research projects funded by the NHS. It contains information on over 28 000 research projects, as well as information from the Medical Research Council's (MRC) Clinical Trials Register, and details of systematic reviews currently in progress from the NHS CRD. It is the most comprehensive register of current NHS research. As such it has great value both as a source of information on unpublished research and also as a way of accessing the full scope of NHS research. The Register uses the MeSH (medical subject heading) thesaurus as an indexing tool.

The NRR can be accessed on the Internet at:

http://www.doh.gov.uk/research/nrr.htm

OMNI (Organising Medical Networked Information Projects)

OMNI is not a database as such; it is a 'gateway'. Gateways (also known as portals or directories) are more sophisticated and rigorous than search engines, although they serve a similar purpose in that they allow access to information available on the Web. Gateways are created by human (rather than computer) searchers. Gateway indexers visit and review Web sites and then catalogue the chosen sites under appropriate subject headings. Gateways can be searched by *browsing* or by *key word searching*. For more information about OMNI see the entry below under Web sites.

OT BibSys

OT BibSys is a database covering both the OT literature and related topic areas such as rehabilitation, education, psychiatry, psychology and health care delivery. It will provide bibliographic information for the material listed. The database is run by AOTA/AOTF (see below under 'Useful addresses and other miscellaneous resources'). All of the material listed in OT BibSys is held at the Wilma L West Library (part of AOTF) and Inter-Library Loan or photocopies can be requested from the Library. The aim of the database is to bring together OT literature into one database. The non-OT specific literature is limited to that written by OTs or of direct interest to OTs. The thesaurus for OT BibSys is based on MeSH (medical subject headings).

OT BibSys is not a free service. There are three subscription categories:

- Individual member (member of AOTA)
- Individual non-member
- Institution

The individual non-member rate is currently US$200 per year.

The OT BibSys Web site is:

http://www.aotf.org/html/ot_bibsys.html

OTDBASE

OTDBASE is a database of OT journal literature. It was developed by a Canadian OT, Marilyn Ernest-Conibear. The database contains abstracts from 17 OT journals and is indexed using 18 OT subject areas, giving some 240 topic areas, with new topic areas being added as the profession develops. Entries are cross-referenced wherever possible to make searching as comprehensive and as simple as possible. The database is updated monthly.

The database can now be accessed in two ways:

- via miniOTDBASE
- by subscription to OTDBASE

MiniOTDBASE is a collaboration between OTDBASE and OT Internet World (see below). It offers free access to a small part of OTDBASE (hence, miniOTDBASE) and so is particularly useful to students and researchers with limited access to institutional resources or on limited budgets. MiniOTDBASE can be accessed on:

http://www.mother.com/~ktherapy/ot

click on the word 'OTDBASEMINI'.

After an introductory paragraph there is a list of key words – such as:

Activity
ADL
Fieldwork
Mental health
OT education
OT research
Orthotics

Click on a key word and you will get a listing of three of the more recent citations linked to these key words.

The value of this service is that it gives the evidence-based practitioner free access to the most recent evidence. It can also help novice searchers to refine their search by highlighting possible key words and allowing them to see whether the chosen key words produce any citations, rather than waste a great deal of time and effort (and possibly, money) on a search that produces nothing.

For access to the full OTDBASE you need to *subscribe* to OTDBASE. This will allow unlimited search access to the whole of OTDBASE. Individual subscription currently costs US$50. You can also subscribe separately to the *OTDBASE UPDATE Newsletter*, a bi-monthly publication containing all the new abstracts of OT journals that have been added to the database.

OTDBASE is only available on-line. However, it does claim to be fast and easy to use. All entries are cross-referenced. Having chosen *one* key term from the main index (e.g. mental health), you are then given a further list of key terms to chose from (e.g. activity, depression); you will then be given a list of all the relevant references in the OTDBASE indexed journals. The beauty of this service is its simplicity. However, this is also its limitation; the *index* supplies the search terms, not the searcher. The other limitation of OTDBASE is that it is a database exclusively of OT literature. Thus, it will not index articles written by OTs, or about OT, but published in non-OT journals. The citations include bibliographic information and the article abstract. OTDBASE claims to be easier to use and to be more comprehensive (in terms of journal information) than OT BibSys. However, OT BibSys includes conference proceedings and other information, which OTDBASE does not.

OTDBASE can be accessed on:

http://www.mother.com/~ktherapy/ot/index1.htm

More information is available from Richard L Powell at:

richardpowell@otdbase.com

PsycLit

PsycLit's focus is psychology and related disciplines, including sociology, anthropology, education, law and medicine. PsycLit indexes over 1300 journals (from 1974) and books (from 1987).

Sociological Abstracts

This database was previously known as SocioFile. It covers sociology and related disciplines. The definition of related disciplines is very broad and includes health and psychology as well as social work, social policy and community care. Over 2000 journals, in 30 languages, from 55 countries are included on this database.

Web sites

This section does not claim to include an exhaustive list of relevant sites. Rather it aims to give an overview of Web sites which the author has found particularly useful or noteworthy. Other Web sites are included within entries in other more relevant sections (e.g. COT Web site, AOTA Web site). A more comprehensive listing of relevant Web sites can by found in Reed and Cunningham (1997).

AOTMH (Association of Occupational Therapists in Mental Health)

Address: 120, Wilton Road
London, SW1V 1JZ
Tel: 0171 233 8322
Fax: 0171 233 7779
E-mail: profbriefings@msn.com
Web site http://www.profbriefings.co.uk/assoc/aotmh.htm

AOTMH was set up in 1994 as a College of Occupational Therapists' Specialist Section, following the merger of four Special Interest Groups:

- Community Mental Health Occupational Therapists' Special Interest Group
- Occupational Therapists Working in Secure Environments
- Special Interest Group on Alcohol and Substance Misuse
- Occupational Therapists Working with the Homeless

Membership of AOTMH is open to all occupational therapists and support workers working with people experiencing mental health problems.

The objectives of AOTMH are:

- To provide support, advice and encouragement to those working in or interested in the field of mental health
- To exchange, share and disseminate information amongst members through a national network
- To provide opportunities for training by holding specialist study days and conferences which are open to all interested members

At the time of writing the AOTMH Web site is under review, but should provide useful links to other mental health Web resources.

COT (College of Occupational Therapists) – See also p.168

There are a range of OT Internet resources, many of which can be accessed from the COT Web site at:

http://www.cot.co.uk/otnet-search.html

Guidelines

This is a UK-based initiative to develop an electronic database of critically-appraised, clinical practice guidelines for health and allied care professionals across the National Health Service (NHS).

http://www.ihs.ox.ac.uk/guidelines/index.html

NARIC (National Rehabilitation Information Center)

This American resource and Web site gives access to various NARIC databases. These include listings of current research covered by the National Institute on Disability and Rehabilitation Research (NIDRR) programme, current and historical (pre-1993) rehabilitation literature and the NARIC Knowledgebase (an information resource). The databases can be searched or browsed, and seem to hold a wide range of potentially useful information.

http://www.naric.com/naric/search

National Guideline Clearinghouse

This American government Web site contains a database of intervention and practice guidelines:

http://www.guideline.gov

Another American source of guideline information is the Agency for Health Care Policy and Research (AHCPR). Their Web site is:

http://text.nlm.nih.gov/ftrs/dbaccess

OCTEP (Occupational Therapy for Elderly People)

OCTEP is the OT special interest section for OTs working with older people. It has a developing Web site at:

http://www.octep.mcmail.com

OMNI Organising Medical Networked Information

The OMNI Project provides a gateway to good-quality Internet resources covering medicine and allied health areas, both in the UK and throughout the world. All resources entered into OMNI are assessed and reviewed against quality guidelines. The resources accessible though OMNI include:

- Education
- Teaching resources
- Databases
- Professional associations
- Books
- Electronic journals
- PAMS (professions allied to medicine) section

OMNI can be accessed at:

http://www.omni.ac.uk

or through another gateway, PINAKES, at:

http://www.hw.ac.uk/libWWW/irn/pinakes/pinakes.html

OMNI's aim is to provide access and search facilities for health professionals using the Internet. OMNI offers training in using the Internet effectively specifically tailored to the needs of the health care community. Information on training courses and downloadable materials can be accessed at:

http://www.omni.ac.uk/training-centre/

and is also available from:

OMNI
Greenfield Medical Library
Queen's Medical Centre
Nottingham, NG7 2UH
Email: help@omni.ac.uk

The monthly newsletter/update can be accessed at:

http://www.omni.ac.uk/general-info/newsletter.html

OMNI can be searched via its *browse* facility, which gives a range of index subheadings to choose from, or via a *key word search*, which can be linked to the MeSH (medical subject heading) thesaurus. OMNI offers access to quality-assessed Web sites on a wide range of medicine-linked topics. As such it is more focused than a general Web site and might be more successful as a search mechanism for evidence than a Web search using a search engine such as AltaVista or Yahoo. (see Chapter 2 for the outcomes of a Web search using AltaVista).

OT Internet World

This American Web site is one of the largest OT Web sites. It has links to a wide range of OT sites and other resources, and is the main access site for OTDBASE. The majority of the information and resources on this Web site are not evidence-based as such, but will provide a useful source of 'expert information'. This site has links to:

- Just OT – which includes a very comprehensive listing of OT Web sites and discussion groups
- OT Schools Listing – this listing is mainly for US OT schools
- OT Internet Directory
- OT ONLINE Newsletter
- Disability information

A new section on research is being developed with the aim of putting abstracts of OT research onto the Net, thus allowing access to unpublished research findings. The URL (Uniform Resource Locator) is:

http://www.mother.com/~ktherapy/ot/

OT Links

This UK-based Web site has comprehensive links to OT relevant sites throughout the world. The site not only includes the links to other Web sites, but comments on the site's clarity and usefulness. As with OT Internet World (above), the information and resources on this site must be viewed as 'expert information' rather than research-based evidence. However, be warned, not all of the Web link addresses are correct which can be frustrating. Links are organised under various headings:

- Location (UK, Europe, etc.)
- Journals
- Individual OTs
- Student links
- Resources
- Miscellaneous

The URL (Uniform Resource Locator) is:

http://www.iop.kcl.ac.uk/home/trust/ot/otlinks.htm

PubMed

PubMed is MEDLINE on the Web. It allows *free* access to the MEDLINE database. It is available at:

http://www4.ncbi.nlm.nih.gov/pubmed

This means that anyone can search MEDLINE via the Internet. However, PubMed can only offer simple searching using one or two key words and the citations provided do not include the article abstracts. PubMed can, however, provide a useful place to begin a search.

The American National Library of Medicine (NLM), who produce PubMed, have also recently launched MEDLINE*plus* which aims to provide an easy to understand resource for the public which includes MEDLINE as well as links to self-help groups and information on clinical trials. MEDLINE*plus* is available at:

http://medlineplus.nlm.nih.gov/medlineplus/

Apart from links to numerous sources, it also has pre-formatted MEDLINE searches on a number of popular topics.

The School of Health and Related Research, at Sheffield University, (ScHARR)

ScHARR is a multi-disciplinary research centre which covers medical, allied health care and social science perspectives on health care. It is part of the Trent Institute of Health Services Research. ScHARR produces a number of evidence-based resources and has an excellent Web site at:

http://www.shef.ac.uk/~scharr/ir/netting.html

which consists of an A-Z guide and introduction to evidence-based practice on the Internet. The site also has links to evidence-based practice tutorials and a range of evidence-based practice-related resources world-wide. Another ScHARR Web site is:

http://www.shef.ac.uk/~scharr/ir/trawling.html

This gives a very comprehensive guide to databases relevant to health care staff which are available on the Internet and offer free access. ScHARR also produces *The ScHARR Guide to Evidence-based Practice* which provides a very comprehensive overview of sources and resources for evidence-based practice (Web sites, databases, journals, etc.) and an evidence-based practice bibliography. The Guide can be downloaded from the ScHARR entry in *Netting the Evidence* or is available in hard copy (price £10, including postage) from:

ScHARR Information Resources
University of Sheffield
Regent Court
30, Regent Street
Sheffield, S1 4DA

The author of *Netting the Evidence, Trawling the Net* and *The ScHARR Guide to Evidence-based Practice* is Andrew Booth:

E-mail: A.Booth@sheffield.ac.uk

Of particular interest to OTs is ScHARR's 'Nursing and Health Care Resources on the Net' Web site:

http://www.shef.ac.uk/~nhcon

This site lists over 1000 Web sites, mailing lists and news groups. The site is intended to provide a browsable and searchable resource for all nurses and health care professionals. The site contains sections on physiotherapy, OT, mental health, etc. It has a UK bias but worldwide coverage. Andrew Booth also created a special link page for the 1997 InFAH study day on *Finding the Evidence* which can be accessed on:

http://www.shef.ac.uk/~scharr/ir/infah.html

This page is aimed specifically towards allied health interests and has many useful evidence-based practice links.

UEBPP (The Unit for Evidence-Based Practice and Policy)

The aim of UEBPP is to promote a multi-disciplinary focus, a qualitative and context-sensitive dimension and a population perspective to evidence-based health care. The Unit is developing a modular MSc course in Evidence-based Practice. The Web site is at:

http://www.ucl.ac.uk/primcare-popsci/uebpp/uebpp.htm

The site lists courses/research projects/Web sites and the series of *British Medical Journal* articles by Tricia Greenhalgh on various aspects of evidence-based medicine (see also Greenhalgh (1997) below).

Information on other Web sites can be found below in the section on 'Useful address and miscellaneous resources'.

E-mail discussion groups

E-mail discussion groups allow groups of people with similar areas of interest to discuss ideas, issues, etc., via the Internet. One person poses a question or makes a comment, and other list members reply. There are a number of discussion groups, a few of which are listed below.

Critical Appraisal Skills Discussion List

E-mail: critical-appraisal-skills@mailbase.ac.uk

This relatively new UK-based list is linked to the CASPInternational network. The aim of the list is to provide a forum for the exchange of information, ideas and experience about finding, critically appraising and using evidence as part of health care delivery. The list is both multi-professional and international in its membership. To join, send the message 'join critical-appraisal-skills *your name*' to mailbase@mailbase.ac.uk.

Evidence-based Health Discussion List

E-mail: evidence-based-medicine@mailbase.ac.uk

This UK-based discussion group is aimed at practitioners and teachers in all health care related areas. The main goal of the group is to assist the implementation of evidence-based health care. The list is also used to debate and discuss issues relevant to evidence-based practice, to announce meetings and courses and to seek information and answers to questions. To join, send the message 'join evidence-based-health *your name*' to mailbase@mailbase.ac.uk.

Occup-ther

E-mail: occup-ther@ac.dal.ca

This Canadian-based OT list is administered by Barbara O'Shea at Dalhousie University. The list is open to qualified OTs only. The list has members throughout the world, although the majority of discussions tend to have a North American slant. However, access to several hundred OTs around the world can provide useful information and ideas about interventions and evidence in OT. To join, send the message 'subscribe occup-ther *your name*' to occup-ther-request@ac.dal.ca.

Occupational-therapy

E-mail: occupational-therapy@mailbase.ac.uk

This is a UK-based OT discussion list. There tends to be considerable overlap between occup-ther and occupational-therapy. UK OTs seem to subscribe and send the same messages to both lists, although non-UK based OTs tend to subscribe to occup-ther. To join, send the message 'join occupational-therapy *your name*' to mailbase@mailbase.ac.uk.

Further reading – books

Bury, T. & Mead, J. (1998) *Evidence-based Healthcare.* Oxford: Butterworth-Heinemann.

This book is aimed at therapists in general. It provides an overview of evidence-based practice and uses case examples to illustrate ideas. It includes some information on finding and appraising evidence. However, its main focus is on implementing change through an evidence-based approach. Its approach is more global than practical. It might be a useful resource for therapy managers and people involved in establishing evidence-based policy at a local level.

Gray, J.A.M (1997) *Evidence-based Healthcare*. Edinburgh: Churchill Livingstone.

This book deals with evidence-based practice from the perspective of policy and management. Gray gives a general introduction to finding and appraising evidence. However, the main focus of the book is on using evidence to develop health care policy and management at local levels and beyond. This is a book for evidence-based managers rather than for evidence-based practitioners.

Greenhalgh, T. (1997) *How to Read a Paper*. London: BMJ Publishing Group.

This book provides a very clear and readable introduction to evidence-based medicine. It includes chapters on finding and appraising a variety of types of published evidence. It is a useful introduction, but the reader must remember that it is written from a *medical* perspective.

Greyson, L. (1997) *Evidence-based Medicine: An Overview and Guide to the Literature*. London: The British Library.

Whilst this book contains some discussion of the nature of evidence-based medicine, its main focus is to provide an overview of the source of literature and other evidence pertinent to an evidence-based approach. As well as reviewing sources of evidence, this book also outlines literature relevant to getting the evidence into practice. Although this book has a more medical focus, it does provide a useful resource for the evidence-based practitioner.

Langhorne, P. & Dennis, M. (1998) *Stroke Units: An Evidence Based Approach*. London: BMJ Publishing Group.

Using the Cochrane Stroke Unit Collaboration systematic review as a basis, this book gives an overview of the role of in-patient stroke units in the care and management of stroke patients. It reviews the evidence for the effectiveness of stroke unit care. The book considers the economics of stroke units and the implications of using the evidence to plan services for stroke patients. This concise volume provides excellent background both to stroke care and to the use of evidence to underpin rehabilitation service delivery.

Li Wan Po, A. (1998) *Dictionary of Evidence-based Medicine*. Abingdon: Radcliffe Medical Press.

An excellent source of definitions of the common terms of evidence-based practice, especially the technical language of biostatistics, epidemiology and health economics. The author has included a number of references for the enthusiastic reader to follow-up discussion of some of the terms and concepts.

Pereira-Maxwell, F. (1998) *A-Z of Medical Statistics: A Companion for Critical Appraisal*. London: Arnold.

This useful little book uses a dictionary format to provide the reader with a succinct overview of medical statistics. It is not intended to be a comprehensive medical statistics textbook. Rather, it provides the evidence-based practitioner with a collection of simple explanations of the key statistical terms and concepts frequently encountered when attempting to read and critically appraise research evidence.

Reed, K.L. & Cunningham, S. (1997) *Internet Guide for Rehabilitation Professionals.* Philadelphia: JB Lippincott Co.

This book is a veritable gold mine of information about the Internet with a specific focus for rehabilitation. The book begins by giving a user-friendly introduction to the Internet and the mysteries of the World Wide Web. It then goes on to outline how to use the Internet effectively and efficiently. However, possibly the most useful part of the book is the guide to rehabilitation resources on the Net. Resources are listed according to professional groups (e.g. OT, physiotherapy), diagnostic/ impairment groups (e.g. AIDS/HIV, cancer, eating disorders) and clinical areas (e.g. biomechanics, neurology, wellness). Each resource is described and the Web address and e-mail address are given. This book should, however, be used bearing two notes of caution in mind:

- The book does have a predominantly American bias
- The Internet is changing so rapidly that this book could become out of date very quickly

Sackett, D.L. Richardson, W.S., Rosenberg, W.M.C. & Haynes, R.B. (1997) *Evidence-based Medicine: How to Practice and Teach EBM*, Edinburgh: Churchill Livingstone.

This pocket-sized book is designed to be an instant resource for evidence-based medicine. It is aimed at doctors and its focus is totally medical. However, it provides useful, basic information about using and teaching evidence-based practice.

Further reading – evidence-based journals and other publications

Bandolier

Bandolier is a newsletter on evidence-based health care, which is produced monthly by the Anglia and Oxford NHS Executive. Its format is bullet points of information about evidence-based medicine, hence the name Bandolier. It is available in print form or via the Internet. Internet access is free, however the most up-to-date version is not usually available. The subscription for the printed version is £30 a year. It is available from:

Pain Relief Clinic
The Churchill Hospital
Headington
Oxford, OX3 7LJ

http://www.jr2.ox.ac.uk:80/Bandolier

This site also has good links to other related and evidence-based sites.

Effective Health Care Bulletins

The *Effective Health Care Bulletins*, which are produced by the NHS Centre for Reviews and Dissemination, are available on the World Wide Web at:

http://www.york.ac.uk/inst/crd/ehcb.htm

They are also available bi-monthly in print form. These bulletins are designed to help health care decision-makers. They examine the effectiveness of various health care interventions. The information in each bulletin is based on systematic reviews and a synthesis of the research on clinical effectiveness, cost effectiveness and acceptability of the particular health care intervention being discussed. Each bulletin is subjected to rigorous peer review. *Effective Health Care Bulletins* should be viewed as excellent sources of information on clinical effectiveness of interventions for the evidence-based OT.

Journals

Clinical Evidence
Evidence-based Child Health
Evidence-based Health Policy and Management
Evidence-based Medicine
Evidence-based Mental Health
Evidence-based Nursing
Focus on Alternative and Complementary Therapies

Books

Bailey, D.M. (1997) *Research for the Health Professional*, 2nd edn. Philadelphia: FA Davis Co.

Chalmers, I. & Altman, D.G. (eds) (1995) *Systematic Reviews*. London: BMJ Publishing Group.

Crombie, I.K. (1996) *Pocket Guide to Critical Appraisal*. London: BMJ Publishing Group.

Crump, B. & Drummond, M.F. (1993) *Evaluating Clinical Evidence: A Handbook for Managers*. London: Longman.

DePoy, E. & Gitlin, L.N. (1994) *Introduction to Research*. St Louis: Mosby.
Dixon, R.A., Munro, J.F. & Silcocks, P.B. (1997) *The Evidence Based Medicine Workbook*. Oxford: Butterworth:Heinemann.
Dunning, M., Abi-Aad, G., Gilbert, D., Gillam, S. & Livett, H. (1998) *Turning Evidence into Everyday Practice*. London: King's Fund.
Entwistle, V., Watts, I.S. & Herring, J.E. (1997) *Information About Health Care Effectiveness*. London: King's Fund.
Grbich, C. (1999) *Qualitative Research in Health*. London: Sage.
Hope, T (1997). *Evidence-based Patient Choice*. London: King's Fund.
Lockett, T. (1997) *Evidence-based and Cost-effective Medicine for the Uninitiated*. London: Radcliffe Medical Press
McQuay, H. & Moore, A. (1998) *An Evidence-based Resource for Pain Relief*. Oxford: Oxford University Press.
Munro, B.H. & Page, E.B. (1993) *Statistical Methods for Health Care Research*. Philadelphia: JB Lippincott Co.
Peckham, M. & Smith, R. (eds) (1996) *Scientific Basis of Health Care*. London: BMJ Publishing Group.
Robson, C. (1993) *Real World Research*. Oxford: Blackwell Publishers.
Sinclair, A. & Dickinson, E. (1998) *Effective Practice in Rehabilitation*. London: King's Fund.

Useful addresses and other miscellaneous resources

AOTA/AOTF (American Occupational Therapy Association/American Occupational Therapy Foundation)

Address: 4720 Montgomery Lane,
PO Box 31220
Bethesda
MD 20824-1220
USA
Tel: 301-652-2682
Fax: 301-652-7711
E-mail: aota@aota.org
aotf@aotf.org

Web site: http://www.aota.org
http://www.aotf.org

AOTA is the professional society for OTs in America. It represents the interests of occupational therapy and occupational therapists in the USA. It produces a number of publications including:

American Journal of Occupational Therapy
OT Practice
OT Week

AOTF is a charitable, scientific, educational and literary organisation which aims to expand and refine the body of knowledge of OT and promote the understanding of the value of occupation. AOTF supports scholarship and research into OT in America. It acts as a resource base for OT, through its own library the Wilma L West Library, and OT BibSys (see above). AOTF publishes the *Occupational Therapy Journal of Research.*

The AOTF Web site contains access to a database of assessments related to OT, a database of rehabilitation organisations in America, a listing of on-line databases relevant to rehabilitation and OT, and links to useful OT and non-OT Web sites.

CAOT (Canadian Association of Occupational Therapists)

Address: CTTC
Suite 3400
1125, Colonel By Drive
Ottawa
Ontario
Canada, K1S 5R1
Tel: (613) 523-2268
Fax: (613) 523-2552
Web site: http://www.caot.ca

CAOT is the professional association for OTs in Canada. In addition to publishing:

Canadian Journal of Occupational Therapy
Occupational Therapy Now

CAOT has been instrumental in the formulation of client-centred practice within OT.

CASP (Critical Appraisal Skills Programme)

Address: Institute of Health Sciences
Old Road
Headington,
Oxford, OX3 7LF
Tel: 01865 226968
Fax: 01865 226959
E-mail: casp@cix.co.uk
Web site: http://www.ihs.ox.ac.uk/casp

CASP's aim is to help health service professionals develop skills in the critical appraisal of evidence about effectiveness and to promote the delivery of evidence-based health care. CASP runs $\frac{1}{2}$ day workshops on the key skills of finding and making sense of evidence to support health care decisions. CASP also runs training the trainer workshops, to help people develop the skills of teaching critical appraisal skills. CASP has recently developed an open learning resource and an interactive CD-ROM on evidence-based health care. The CASP Web site has links to a variety of useful Web sites.

The CASPInternational network has recently been established to share and promote good practice in finding and appraising evidence throughout the world. CASPInternational's Web site is:

http://phru.org/caspinternational/

E-mail: pbradley@demon.co.uk

The CASPInternational co-ordinator is:
Peter Bradley
Highfield Northamptonshire Health Authority

Cliftonville Road
Northampton, NN1 5DN
Tel: 01604 615208
Fax: 01604 615146

Centre for Evidence-Based Medicine (CEBM)

Address: NHS R&D Centre for Evidence-Based Medicine
Oxford Radcliffe NHS Trust
Headley Way
Headington
Oxford, OX3 9DU
Tel: 01865 222941
Fax: 01865 222901
Web site: http://cebm.jr2.ox.ac.uk

The CEBM was opened in March 1995 and is based at the John Radcliffe Hospital in Oxford. Its remit is:

- To promote the teaching and practice of evidence-based health care throughout the UK
- To effect the creation of formal graduate education in the conduct of randomised controlled trials and systematic reviews in the University of Oxford.

Although its focus is predominantly medical, the CEBM is a valuable resource for the evidence-based OT. The CEBM Web site is well worth a visit, as it contains teaching resources as well as useful links to other evidence-based Web sites.

Centre for Evidence-Based Mental Health

Address: Department of Psychiatry
University of Oxford
Warneford Hospital
Oxford, OX3 7JX

Tel: 01865 226480
Fax: 01865 793101
Web site: http://www.psychiatry.ox.ac.uk/cebmh/

This is a useful resource for all mental health practitioners. The Web site contains a range of resources for teaching and using an evidence-based approach within mental health settings. OXAMWEB at:

http://www.psychiatry.ac.uk/cebmh/oxamweb/

has excellent links to evidence-based mental health sites. It aims to give users access to high-quality evidence in *less than three clicks* by using key words to allow access to evidence-based information on the Internet.

Centre for Evidence-Based Nursing

Address: University of York
York, YO10 5DQ

Centre for Evidence-Based Social Services

Address: University of Exeter
Amory Building
Rennes Drive
Exeter, EX4 4RJ
Tel: 01392 263 323
Fax: 01392 263 324
Web site: http://www.ex.ac.uk/cebss/

COT (College of Occupational Therapists)

Address: 106–114 Borough High Street
Southwark
London, SE1 1LB
Tel: 020 7357 6480
Fax: 020 7250 2299

Web sites: http://www.cot.co.uk
http://www.baot.co.uk

The College of Occupational Therapists (COT) is the professional body for OTs in the UK. The College of Occupational Therapists also has a Library and Information Service which is available to members. This service can be accessed by telephone, fax, written query, e-mail or visited in person. The library holds a collection of OT journals as well as a thesis and dissertation collection. There are reference facilities including CINAHL and AMED. The library produces Current Awareness Bulletins and factsheets. They can provide photocopies of reference material, and dissertations and theses can be borrowed from the library.

The address of the library is the same as COT (above)

Tel: 020 7450 2316
Fax: 020 7450 2299

NHS CRD (NHS Centre for Reviews and Dissemination)

Address: University of York
Heslington
York, YO1 5DD
Tel: 01904 433643
Fax: 01904 433661
Web site: http://www.york.ac.uk/inst/crd/

The NHS CRD is commissioned by the NHS R&D Directorate to produce and disseminate reviews concerning the effectiveness and cost effectiveness of health care interventions. The aim of NHS CRD is to identify and review the results of good-quality health research and to disseminate actively the findings to key decision-makers in the NHS and to consumers of health care services. In this way health care professionals and managers can ensure their practice reflects the best available research evidence. The reviews cover: the effectiveness of care for particular conditions; the effectiveness of health technologies; evidence on efficient methods of organising and delivering particular types of health care. The reviews are collected into a database of structured abstracts of good-quality systematic reviews (DARE) which comment on the methodological features of published reviews and summarise the author's conclusions and any implications for health practice. The abstracts represent the end-product of a detailed sifting and quality appraisal process.

UK Cochrane Centre

Address: NHS Research and Development Programme
Summertown Pavilion
Middle Way
Oxford, OX2 7LG
Tel: 01865 516300
Fax: 01865 516311
Web site: http://www.hiru/mcmaster.ca/cochrane/centres/UK/

University of Oxford Department of Continuing Education

Address: 1, Wellington Square
Oxford, OX1 2JA
Tel: 01865 280347
Fax: 01865 270386
E-mail: elaine.welsh@conted.ox.ac.uk

The University of Oxford's Centre for Continuing Professional Development runs the Oxford Master's Programme in Evidence-Based Health Care. The programme is modular and part-time. It consists of three related courses:

- Postgraduate Certificate
- Postgraduate Diploma
- MSc

The programme is aimed at professionals working in any area of health care.

GLOSSARY

AMED is the Allied and Alternative Medicine database and as such provides a useful source of references of specific relevance to the evidence-based OT (see Chapters 2 and 7).

ASSIA (Applied Social Science Index of Abstracts) is a key source for social science references, with good coverage of applied social care topics (see Chapters 2 and 7).

Bandolier is a monthly newsletter, published by the Anglia and Oxford NHS Executive. It focuses on evidence-based practice and gives brief overviews of relevant issues (see Chapter 7).

Bias refers to the systematic deviation of results from the true value of the results. There are two main sources of bias in intervention research:

- Poor sampling, which will lead to non-representative groups of participants being used in a study
- Problems with the actual process of the study or the measurement tools used in the study.

Blind refers to the fact that the researchers and/or the participants were unaware of which experimental group the participant was in. This ensures that the researcher and/or the participant are not influenced by knowing that they are in the **experimental group** or the **control group**.

- **Single blind** studies are where the participants are unaware of which intervention they are receiving.
- **Double blind** studies are where both the participants and the health professionals administering the interventions are unaware of whether the participant is part of the intervention group or the control group.

Boolean operators are words such as AND, OR and NOT which are used to refine search terms when carrying out literature searches (see Chapter 2).

CASP (Critical Appraisal Skills Programme) runs workshops to help practitioners develop their critical appraisal skills. They also produce distance learning packs and a **CD-ROM** to help practitioners to refine their evidence-based skills (see Chapter 7).

CCT see **controlled clinical trial**.

CD-ROM (Compact Disc-Read Only Memory) is a compact disc which has data stored on it; this data can be read by a computer but cannot be changed by the computer. Databases, such as the **Cochrane Library**, are available in CD-ROM format.

CI see **confidence interval**.

CINAHL (Cumulative Index of Nursing and Allied Health Literature) is a database of predominantly nursing literature with some rehabilitation and allied health literature (see Chapters 2 and 7).

Clinical effectiveness is the extent to which a particular intervention/procedure/service improves the outcome for the clients as opposed to **efficacy** which refers to the ideal or restricted parameters of a **randomised controlled trial**. Clinical effectiveness is also known simply as **effectiveness**.

Clinical governance is the philosophy and framework through which National Health Service (NHS) organisations are accountable for continuously assessing and improving the quality of the services they provide.

Clinical guidelines are systematically developed statements which are aimed to help practitioners and clients make rational decisions about the most appropriate health care for specific problems.

Clinical significance is seen in terms of the size of the treatment effect and is expressed in terms of **odds ratios** and **numbers needed to treat**. Deciding how large the treatment effect should be before an intervention is seen as clinically significant is a matter of practitioner judgement. Studies may be **statistically significant** without being clinically significant.

Cochrane Collaboration is a collaborative network focusing on carrying out, and making accessible, systematic reviews of **randomised controlled trials** of health care. The collaboration began with the establishment of the

UK Cochrane Centre but the collaboration is now international with a number of national centres co-ordinating the work of review groups and networks. The main output of the collaboration is the **Cochrane Library**.

Cochrane Library is a quarterly publication (on disk/CD-ROM and Internet access) produced by the **Cochrane Collaboration**. It consists of four separate databases:

- The Cochrane Database of Systematic Reviews
- The York Database of Abstracts of Reviews of Effectiveness (**DARE**)
- The Cochrane Controlled Trials Register
- The Cochrane Review Methodology Database.

(see Chapter 7 for more information).

Confidence interval (CI) is the range of values within which the 'true' result can be found, with a given level of confidence. Commonly accepted confidence intervals are 95% or 99%. This means that the true result lies somewhere between the two given values in 95% (or 99%) of cases (see Chapter 3).

Confirmability refers to the strategies used by qualitative researchers to limit **bias** within their research (see Chapter 5).

Controlled clinical trial (CCT) is a trial where interventions are compared, as in a **randomised controlled trial**, but where it is not possible (for practical or ethical reasons) to randomly (see **randomisation**) allocate the participants to the various study groups (see Chapter 3).

Controls or the **control group**, are the participants in a **randomised controlled trial** who provide the comparison group. They receive the standard intervention (or a **placebo**, or no intervention) so that their outcomes can be compared to those of the experimental group in order to access the **efficacy** of the intervention under trial.

Credibility is used to assess the **rigour** of qualitative research. It refers to whether the research is giving a true picture of the phenomenon being studied. A good test of credibility is whether the descriptions and interpretations of the phenomenon being researched are recognisable to people outside the research setting (see Chapter 5).

Critical appraisal is the process of reviewing, assessing and interpreting evidence by systematically considering its **rigour**, results and its relevance to your own area of practice (see also **CASP**).

DARE (Database of Abstracts of Reviews of Effectiveness) is produced by the NHS Centre for Reviews and Dissemination (NHS CRD) at York University. It is a database of quality-assessed **systematic reviews** and as such is a valuable source of high-quality evidence for the evidence-based OT (see Chapter 7).

Dependability is another technique for assessing the **rigour** of a piece of qualitative research. It relates to how consistent the data and findings of the study are (see Chapter 5).

Effectiveness see **clinical effectiveness**.

Efficacy is the extent to which an intervention improves the outcome for patients under ideal circumstances.

Ethnography is a method of qualitative research. The main focus of ethnographic studies is the exploration of cultures (see Chapter 5).

Experimental group (or condition) is the group of participants, in a **randomised controlled trial** (RCT) who received the new intervention. If the outcome for this group is better, in comparison to the **control group**, the RCT can be seen as providing evidence for the **efficacy** of the intervention.

Free text searching is when natural (or everyday) language and terms are used as the search terms in a literature search.

Generalisability is a term used especially within quantitative research to indicate how well the results of one study can be applied to a more general population.

Gold standard refers to what is generally regarded as the best available evidence, method or measure. In evidence-based practice **randomised controlled trials** are seen as the gold standard for evidence, against which all other research is compared and found wanting.

Heterogeneity refers to *differences* in results or participant groups. Heterogeneity is often assessed in **systematic reviews** and **meta-analyses**, when the results for the various studies appear to be markedly different. If there is evidence of heterogeneity, a single summary of the individual results within a review should not be given. Systematic reviews often include tests of heterogeneity, however these tests are not very powerful and can be confusing. Individual judgement and appraisal is probably the best assessment of heterogeneity. The opposite of heterogeneity is **homogeneity**.

Homogeneity is a measure of the *similarity* of a group of research participants or results. Studies are said to be homogeneous if the spread of their results is less than would be expected as chance variations. Homogenous subject (or participant) groups are groups of people who are similar along the defined parameters of the study (e.g. age, gender, social class, diagnosis, length of intervention). The opposite of homogeneity is **heterogeneity**.

Hypothesis is a testable statement, usually stating a cause and effect, which is the basis of experimental (and **randomised controlled trial**) research.

Mean is the average value for a particular group of data. It is calculated by adding together all of the measurements (scores) and dividing them by the number of measurements (participants).

Median is the value on a scale, or series of data, that indicates the midpoint in the data set. Half of the observations (scores) are below this number and the other half are above this number.

MEDLINE is a database of biomedical literature. It is the largest and most popular medical database. It is available by subscription on **CD-ROM**. The (free) on-line version of MEDLINE is **PubMed**. (see Chapter 7).

MeSH (medical subject heading) is the indexing system used by **MEDLINE** and other health/medical orientated database systems.

Meta-analysis is a statistical technique used predominantly in **systematic reviews** which summarises the results of a number of studies into one estimate of the **efficacy** of an intervention.

NICE (National Institute of Clinical Excellence) has been set up by the Department of Health to promote clinical cost effectiveness and the production and dissemination of **clinical guidelines**.

NNT see **numbers needed to treat**.

Numbers needed to treat (NNT) is used as a measure of the **clinical effectiveness** of a treatment, and the **clinical significance** of a **systematic review**. The NNT is the number of people who would need to be treated with a specific intervention (e.g. admission to a stroke unit) to produce an occurrence of a specific outcome (e.g. prevention of death or dependency).

Odds ratio (OR) is a measure of an intervention's **clinical effectiveness** and **clinical significance**. It refers to the likelihood of the experimental intervention being effective in comparison to the control intervention. An odds ratio of 1 indicates that there is the same likelihood (odds) of the outcome occurring in both the intervention and the control group. An odds ratio of *less than* 1 indicates a better outcome in the intervention group, or evidence for the effectiveness of the intervention. An odds ratio of *more than* 1 indicates better outcomes in the control group, or no evidence for the effectiveness of the intervention (see Chapter 4).

OMNI is an Internet 'gateway' which gives access to Web sites of interest to medical practitioners (see Chapter 7).

OR see **odds ratio**.

OT BibSys is a database covering both the OT literature and related topic areas such as rehabilitation, education, psychiatry, psychology and health care delivery. It will provide bibliographic information for the material listed. The database is run by AOTA/AOTF (see Chapter 7).

OTDBASE is a database of OT journal literature. It is available on-line by subscription (see Chapters 2 and 7).

Phenomenology is a qualitative research method. The main focus of phenomenological research is understanding the experience of a particular event (phenomenon) from the perspective of the participant.

Placebo is an inactive treatment often given as part of **a randomised controlled trial**. The placebo intervention is delivered in a way that makes it appear identical to the experimental intervention as a way of eliminating any psychological effects on participants of being in a study.

Probability refers to the likelihood of any result occurring due to chance factors as opposed to due to the effect of the intervention (see Chapter 3).

Publication bias can result if only studies indicating positive or successful findings are published. However, the tendency for journals to only publish 'significant' research is changing. Critical appraisers of **systematic reviews** should be aware that only positive research might be published or chosen for a review.

PubMed is the (free) on-line version of **MEDLINE** (see Chapters 2 and 7).

Randomisation is the process of allocating participants to various groups within a **randomised controlled trial**. Each participant has the same likelihood of being allocated to the experimental condition as the control condition. Randomisation is carried out as a way of ensuring that all participant groups are as similar as possible in terms of key variables (e.g. age, sex, social class) (see Chapter 3).

Randomised controlled trial (RCT) is a study of the effectiveness of an intervention where the participants have been randomly (see **randomisation**) allocated to the various groups (e.g. experimental, control, alternative intervention) (see **controlled clinical trial** and Chapter 3).

RCT see **randomised controlled trial**.

Reliability is a measure of the **rigour** of a piece of quantitative research. Reliability implies that the study would give the same results if the measures used were repeated, either by the same researcher or by other researchers.

Review is any summary of the literature on a particular topic. It may include research and non-research literature and may not have attempted to ensure that all literature is accessed or that the quality of the research is assessed, in contrast to a **systematic review**.

Rigour refers to whether a piece of research has been conducted to ensure that any **bias** is reduced to a minimum, that the research has as much **validity/reliability/trustworthiness** as possible and that the appropriate techniques and strategies have been used to ensure this.

Statistical significance refers to the result of a statistical test, when the associated *P*-value (see also **probability)** is found to be below a predetermined cut-off point, conventionally set at $P = 0.05$. Statistical significance is often written as '$P < 0.05$', however with modern computer statistical packages it is possible to calculate the exact *P*-value and this should be stated (see Chapter 3).

Systematic review is a review and synthesis of the research literature on a particular topic. A systematic review will attempt to access ALL published and unpublished literature on the chosen topic. Studies are only included in the review if they meet pre-determined criteria of research quality. The findings of the various studies may be combined using **meta-analysis**, if appropriate (see Chapter 4).

Transferability is a way of assessing the **rigour** of qualitative research. It refers to how well the research achieves 'goodness of fit' with other contexts. It is the task of the appraiser (rather than the researcher) to decide how transferable a piece of research is (see Chapter 5).

Triangulation is a strategy for ensuring **rigour** in qualitative research. It involves collecting data from a number of different sources and utilising a number of different data collection techniques. (see Chapter 5).

Trustworthiness refers to the **rigour** of a piece of qualitative research. Aspects of trustworthiness in qualitative research include:

Confirmability, Credibility, Dependability and Transferability (see Chapter 5).

Validity refers to the **rigour** of a piece of quantitative research. A study is valid if it does what it set out to do and if the measures used actually measure what they purport to measure.

REFERENCES

American Occupational Therapy Association (1996) *Occupational Therapy Practice Guidelines for Adults with Stroke*. Bethesda: American Occupational Therapy Association.

Arnold, C., Bain, J., Brown, R. (1995) *Moving to Audit: An Education Package for the Professions Allied to Medicine*. Dundee: Centre for Medical Education.

Austin, C. & Herbert, S.I. (1995) Clinical guidelines: should we be worried? *British Journal of Occupational Therapy*, **58**(11), 481–4.

Bailey, D.M. (1991) *Research for the Health Professional*. Philadelphia: FA Davis Co.

Bailey, D.M. (1997) *Research for the Health Professional*, 2nd edn. Philadelphia: FA Davis Co.

Baker, R., Dowling, Z., Wareing, L.A., Dawson, J. & Assey, J. (1997). Snoezelen: its long-term effects on older people with dementia. *British Journal of Occupational Therapy*, **60**(5), 213–18.

Bennett, K.J., Sackett, D.L., Haynes, R.B., Neufeld, V.R., Tugwell, P. & Roberts, R. (1987) A controlled trial of teaching critical appraisal of the clinical literature to medical students. *Journal of the American Medical Association*, **257**(18), 2451–4.

British Journal of Therapy & Rehabilitation (1996) Supplement on evidence-based practice and mental health. *British Journal of Therapy and Rehabilitation*, **3**(12), 659–70.

Brown, G.T. (1998) Research utilization: a purposeful activity for occupational therapists. Paper presentation, *12th International Congress of the World Federation of Occupational Therapists*, Montreal.

Bury, T. (1998) Getting research into practice: changing behaviour. In: *Evidence-based Healthcare*, (eds T. Bury & J. Mead), pp. 66–84. Oxford: Butterworth-Heinemann.

Buttery, Y. (1998) Implementing evidence through clinical audit. In: *Evidence-based Healthcare*, (eds T. Bury & J. Mead), pp. 182–207. Oxford: Butterworth-Heinemann.

Canadian Association of Occupational Therapists (1991) *Occupational Therapy Guidelines for Client-centred Practice.* Toronto: Canadian Association of Occupational Therapists.

Canadian Association of Occupational Therapists (1997) *Enabling Occupation: An Occupational Therapy Perspective.* Ottawa: Canadian Association of Occupational Therapists.

Canadian Association of Occupational Therapists (1998) Special edition on evidence-based practice. *Canadian Journal of Occupational Therapy,* **65**(3).

Canadian Task Force on the Periodic Health Examination (1979) The periodic health examination. *Canadian Medical Association Journal*, **121**, 1193–254.

Carlson, M., Fanchiang, S.P., Zemke, R. & Clark, F. (1996) A meta-analysis of the effectiveness of occupational therapy for older persons. *American Journal of Occupational Therapy*, **50**(2), 89–98.

Chartered Society of Physiotherapy (1996) *Literature Searching: Where to Go and What to Look For.* London: Chartered Society of Physiotherapy.

Clark, F., Azen, A.P., Zemke, R. *et al.* (1997) Occupational therapy for independent living older adults. *Journal of the American Medical Association* **278**(16), 1321–6.

Clemence, M.L. (1998) Evidence-base physiotherapy: seeking the unattainable? *British Journal of Therapy and Rehabilitation*, **5**(5), 257–60.

Cochrane, A. (1972) *Effectiveness & Efficiency.* London: Nuffield Provincial Hospitals Trust.

College of Occupational Therapists (1990) *Guidelines for Documentation*. London: College of Occupational Therapists.

College of Occupational Therapists, (1995) *Code of Ethics and Professional Conduct for Occupational Therapists.* London: College of Occupational Therapists.

College of Occupational Therapists (1997) Special edition on evidence-based practice. *British Journal of Occupational Therapy*, **60**(11).

Cooper, E.J. (1995) *Does the Rivermead Extended ADL Score Indicate a Patient's Level of Independence After Discharge?* Unpublished dissertation: Oxford Brookes University.

Cusick, A. (1986) Research in occupational therapy: meta-analysis. *Australian Occupational Therapy Journal*, **33**(4), 142–7.

Dale, P. (ed.) (1997) *Guide to Libraries and Information Sources in Medicine and Health Care*. London: The British Library.

Denzin, N.K. & Lincoln, Y.S. (1994) Introduction: Entering the field of qualitative research. In: *Handbook of Qualitative Research*, (eds N.K. Denzin & Y.S. Lincoln), pp. 1–17. Thousand Oaks: Sage.

Department of Health (1991) PL/CNO (91/3). *Audit for Nursing and Therapy Professions in HCHS: Allocation of Funds 1991/92*. London: Department of Health.

Department of Health (1997) *The New NHS: Modern – Dependable*. London: HMSO.

DePoy, E. & Gitlin, L.N. (1994) *Introduction to Research*. St Louis: Mosby.

Droogan, J. & Bannigan, K. (1997) A review of psychosocial family interventions for schizophrenia. *Nursing Times*, **93**(26), 46–7.

Dunning, M., Abi-Aad, G., Gilbert, D., Gillam, S. & Livett, H. (1998) *Turning Evidence into Everyday Practice*. London: King's Fund.

Eysenck, H.J. (1978) An exercise in mega-silliness. *American Psychologist*, **33**, 517.

Finlay, L. (1997) Good patients and bad patients: how occupational therapists view their patients/clients. *British Journal of Occupational Therapy*, **60**(10), 440–46.

Finlay, L (1998). Reflexivity: an essential component of all research? *British Journal of Occupational Therapy*, **61**(10), 453–6.

Gray, J.A.M. (1997) *Evidence-based Healthcare*. Edinburgh: Churchill Livingstone.

Greenhalgh, T. (1997) *How to Read a Paper*. London: BMJ Publishing Group.

Greyson, L. (1997) *Evidence-based Medicine: An Overview and Guide to the Literature*. London: The British Library.

Haddon-Silver, A. (1993) *Homophobia Amongst OT Students: Issues, Incidence and Implications*. Unpublished dissertation: Oxford Brookes University.

Hasselkus, B.R. (1992) The meaning of activity: day care for persons with Alzheimer disease. *American Journal of Occupational Therapy*, **46**, 199–206.

Helm, T. & Dickerson, A.E. (1995) The effect of hand therapy on a patient with a Colles' fracture: a phenomenological study. *Occupational Therapy in Health Care*, **9**(4), 69–77.

Keep, J (1998) Change management. In: *Evidence-based Healthcare*, (eds T. Bury & J. Mead), pp. 45–65. Oxford: Butterworth-Heinemann.

Kielhofner, G. (1982). Qualitative research: part two, methodological approaches and relevance to occupational therapy. *Occupational Therapy Journal of Research*, **2**, 150–70.

Kogan, M., Redfern, S., Kober, A. *et al.* (1995) *Making Use of Clinical Audit: A Guide to Practice in the Health Professions.* Buckingham: Open University Press.

Krefting, L.M. (1989a) Disability ethnography: a methodological approach for occupational therapy. *Canadian Journal of Occupational Therapy*, **56**(2), 61–6.

Krefting, L.M. (1989b) Reintegration into the community after head injury: the results of an ethnographic study. *Occupational Therapy Journal of Research*, **9**, 67–83.

Krefting, L.M. (1991) Rigor in qualitative research: the assessment of trustworthiness. *American Journal of Occupational Therapy*, **45**(3), 214–22.

Langhorne, P. & Dennis, M. (1998) *Stroke Units: An Evidence Based Approach*. London: BMJ Publishing Group.

Langhorne, P., Wagenaar, R. & Partridge, C. (1996) Physiotherapy after stroke: more is better? *Physiotherapy Research International*, **1**(2), 75–88.

Law, M. (ed.) (1998) *Client-centered Occupational Therapy.* Thorofare, NJ: Slack.

Li Wan Po, A. (1998) Dictionary of Evidence-based Medicine. Abingdon: Radcliffe Press.

Liddle, J., March, L., Carfrae, B. *et al.* (1996) Can occupational therapy intervention play a part in maintaining independence and quality of life in older people? A randomised controlled trial. *Australian and New Zealand Journal of Public Health*, **20**(6), 574–8.

Lin, K., Wu, C., Tickle-Degnen, L. & Coster, W. (1997) Enhancing occupational performance through occupationally embedded exercise: a meta-analytic review. *Occupational Therapy Journal of Research*, **17**(1), 25–47.

Lincoln, Y.S. & Guba, E.A. (1985) *Naturalistic Inquiry.* Beverly Hills: Sage.

Linzer, M. (1987) The journal club and medical education: over one hundred years of unrecorded history. *Postgraduate Medical Journal*, **63**, 475–8.

Linzer, M., Brown, T., Frazier, L. *et al.* (1988) Impact of a medical journal on house-staff reading habits, knowledge and critical appraisal skills. *Journal of the American Medical Association*, **260**, 2537–41.

Littlewood, S.A. (1997) *Do OT Students Consider Sexual Orientation When Implementing Treatment.* Unpublished dissertation: Oxford Brookes University.

Logan, P.A., Ahern, J., Gladman, J.R. & Lincoln, N.B. (1997) A randomized controlled trial of enhanced Social Services occupational therapy for stroke patients. *Clinical Rehabilitation*, **11**(2), 107–13.

McCuaig, M. & Frank, G. (1991) The able self: adaptive patterns and choices in independent living for a person with cerebral palsy. *American Journal of Occupational Therapy*, **45**(3), 224–34.

McKinnell, I. & Elliott, J. (1997) *The Cochrane Library: Self-Training Guide and Notes.* Oxford: Anglia and Oxford. NHS Executive. http://www.lib.jr2.ox.ac.uk/nhserdd/aordd/evidence/clibtrng.htm

Malby, R. (1995) *Clinical Audit for Nurses and Therapists.* London: Scutari.

Mann, T. (1996) *Clinical Guidelines: Using Clinical Guidelines to Improve Patient Care within the NHS.* London: Department of Health.

Mattingly, C. & Fleming, M.H. (1994) *Clinical Reasoning: Forms of Inquiry in a Therapeutic Practice*. Philadelphia: FA Davis Co.

Moreton, S (1998). Local clinical guidelines – can they make us better? Paper presentation, *12th International Congress of the World Federation of Occupational Therapists*, Montreal.

Mulrow, C.D. (1994) Rationale for systematic reviews. *British Medical Journal*, **309**, 597–9.

Mulrow, C.D. & Oxman, A.D. (eds) (1997) *Cochrane Collaboration Handbook* [updated September, 1997]. In: The Cochrane Library [database on disk and CD-ROM]. The Cochrane Collaboration. Oxford: Update Software; 1994, issue 4.

Munro, B.H. & Page, E.B. (1993) *Statistical Methods for Health Care Research*. Philadelphia: JB Lippincott Co.

Munroe, H. (1996) Clinical reasoning in community occupational therapy. *British Journal of Occupational Therapy*, **59**(5), 196–202.

Needham, G. & Oliver, S. (1998) Involving service users. In: *Evidence-based Healthcare*, (eds T. Bury & J. Mead), pp. 85–104. Oxford: Butterworth-Heinemann.

Newell, R. (1997) Towards clinical effectiveness in nursing. *Clinical Effectiveness Nursing*, **1**(1), 1–2.

NHS Executive (1996) *Promoting Clinical Effectiveness: A Framework for Action*. Leeds: NHS Executive.

NHS Executive (1998) *Information for Health: An Information Strategy for the Modern NHS 1998–2005. A National Strategy for Local Implementation*. Leeds/London: Department of Health.

NHS Management Executive (1994) EL(94)20. *Clinical Audit: 1994/95 and Beyond*. London: Department of Health.

Occupational Therapy for Elderly People, (1997) *OCTEP Newsletter*. Autumn, 1997.

Ottenbacher, K. (1983) Quantitative reviewing: the literature review as scientific inquiry. *American Journal of Occupational Therapy*, **37**(5), 313-19.

Pereira-Maxwell, F. (1998) *A–Z of Medical Statistics: A Companion for Critical Appraisal*. London: Arnold.

Piercy, M. (1998) *An Audit of the Reliability of the Frenchay Activities Index*. Unpublished dissertation: Oxford Brookes University.

Popay, J., Rogers, A. & Williams, G. (1998) Rationale and standards for the systematic review of qualitative literature in health services research. *Journal of Qualitative Health Research*, **8**, 341–51.

Popay, J. & Williams, G. (1998) Qualitative research and evidence-based healthcare. *Journal of the Royal Society of Medicine*, **91**(Suppl. 35), 32–7.

Przybylski, B.R., Dumont, E.D., Watkins, M.E., Warren, S.A., Beaulne, A.P. & Lier, D.A. (1996) Outcomes of enhanced physical and occupational therapy service in a nursing home setting. *Archives of Physical Medicine and Rehabilitation*, **77**(6), 554–61.

Rangachari, P.K. (1997) Evidence-based medicine: old French wine with a new Canadian label? *Journal of the Royal Society of Medicine*, **90**, 280–84.

Reed, K.L. & Cunningham, S. (1997) *Internet Guide for Rehabilitation Professionals*. Philadelphia: JB Lippincott Co.

Reynard, K.W. & Reynard, J.M.E. (eds) (1996) *ASLIB Directory of Information Sources in the United Kingdom*. London: ASLIB.

Richardson, W.S., Wilson, M.C., Nishikawa, J. *et al.* (1995) The well-built clinical question: a key to evidence-based decisions (editorial). *ACP Journal Club*, **123**, A12–A13.

Rosenberg, W. & Donald, A. (1995) Evidence based medicine: an approach to clinical problem-solving. *British Medical Journal*, **310**, 1122–6.

Sackett, D. (1997) What is evidence-based practice? Paper presentation. OXRIG: Oxford.

Sackett, D.L., Richardson, W.S., Rosenberg, W.M.C. & Hayes, R.B. (1997) *Evidence-based Medicine: How to Practice and Teach EBM.* New York: Churchill Livingstone.

Sackett, D.L., Rosenberg, W.M.C., Gray, J.A.M., Haynes, R.B. & Richardson, W.S. (1996) Evidence-based medicine: what it is and what it isn't. *British Medical Journal*, **312**, 71–2.

Sale, D. (1996) *Quality Assurance for Nurses and Other Members of the Health Care Team.* London: Macmillan.

Sanford, M.K., Hazelwood, S.E., Bridges, A.J. *et al.* (1996). Effectiveness of computer-assisted interactive videodisc instruction in teaching rheumatology to physical and occupational therapy students. *Journal of Allied Health*, **25**, 141–8.

Schön, D. (1983) *The Reflective Practitioner*. New York: Basic.

Shin, J.H., Haynes, R.B. & Johnston, M.E. (1993) Effect of problem-based, self-directed undergraduate education on life-long learning. *Canadian Medical Association Journal*, **148**(6); 969–76.

Shopland, A.J., Hardial, P.M., Unwin, A.M., Vickers, S.M., Westmore, V.R. & Williams, A.J. (1975) *Refer to Occupational Therapy*. Edinburgh: Churchill Livingstone.

Simpson, J.M., Marsh, N. & Harrington, R. (1998) Guidelines for managing falls among elderly people. *British Journal of Occupational Therapy*, **61**(4), 165–8.

Spector, A. & Orrell, M. (1998a) Reality Orientation for dementia: a review of the evidence of effectiveness (Cochrane Review). In: The Cochrane Library, Issue 3, 1998. Oxford: Update Software.

Spector, A. & Orrell, M. (1998b) Reminiscence Therapy for dementia: a review of the evidence of effectiveness (Cochrane Review). In: The Cochrane Library, Issue 3, 1998. Oxford: Update Software.

Spencer, J., Young, M., Rintala, D. & Bates, S. (1995) Socialization to the culture of a rehabilitation hospital: an ethnographic study. *American Journal of Occupational Therapy*, **49**(1), 53–62.

Sumsion, T. (1997) Client-centred implications of evidence-based practice. *Physiotherapy*, **83**(7), 373–4.

Taylor, M.C. (1997) What is evidence-based practice? *British Journal of Occupational Therapy*, **60**(11), 470–74.

Taylor, M.C. (1999) The devil makes work for idle hands – reviewing the evidence for the value of 'activity' as an intervention for depression. Conference presentation, *2nd Evidence-based Mental Health Conference*, Norwich.

Taylor, L.P. & McGruder, J.E. (1996) The meanings of sea kayaking for persons with spinal cord injuries. *American Journal of Occupational Therapy*, **50**(1), 39–46.

Thomas, L., Cullum, N., McColl, E., Rousseau, N., Soutter, J. & Steen N. (1999) Clinical guidelines in nursing, midwifery and other professions allied to medicine (Cochrane Review). In: *The Cochrane Library*, Issue 1, 1999. Oxford: Update Software.

Townsend, E. (1996) Institutional ethnography: a method of showing how the context shapes practice. *Occupational Therapy Journal of Research*, **16**(3), 179–99.

Turner, P.A. & Whitefield, T.W. (1996) A multivariate analysis of physiotherapy clinicians' journal readership. *Physiotherapy Theory & Practice*, **12**(4), 221–30.

Turner, P. & Whitefield, T.W. (1997) Journal readership amongst Australian physiotherapists: a cross-national replication. *Australian Journal of Physiotherapy*, **43**(3), 197–202.

Upton, D. (1999a) Clinical effectiveness and EBP 2: attitudes of healthcare professionals. *British Journal of Therapy and Rehabilitation*, **6**(1), 26–30.

Upton, D. (1999b) Clinical effectiveness and EBP 3: application by healthcare professionals. *British Journal of Therapy and Rehabilitation*, **6**(2), 86–90.

de Vet, H.C.W., de Bie, R.A., van der Heijden, G.J.M.G., Verhagen, A.P., Sijpkes, P. & Knipschild, P.G. (1997) Systematic reviews on the basis of methodological criteria. *Physiotherapy*, **83**(6), 284–98.

Walshe, K. (1998) Quality moves to the top of the agenda. *Health Service Management Centre Newsletter*, **4**, 2.

Whiteford, G.E. (1998) Intercultural OT: learning, reflection and transformation. *British Journal of Therapy and Rehabilitation*, **5**(6), 299–305.

Wiles, R. & Barnard, S. (1998) Physiotherapy and evidence-based practice. Paper presentation, *British Sociological Association Medical Sociology Group, 30th Annual Conference*: York.

Wilson-Barnett, J (1998). Evidence for nursing practice – an overview. *NT Research*, **3**(1), 12–14.

Yerxa, E.J. (1991) Seeking a relevant, ethical, and realistic way of knowing for occupational therapy. *American Journal of Occupational Therapy*, **45**(3), 199–204.

Zisselman, M.H., Rovner, B.W., Shmuely, Y. & Ferrie, P. (1996). A pet therapy intervention with geriatric inpatients. *American Journal of Occupational Therapy*, **50**(1), 47–51.

INDEX